Essential Oils for Beginners

Essential Oils for Beginners

The Complete Guide to Getting Started with Essential Oils and Aromatherapy

Julia Grady

Copyright © 2014 by Dylanna Publishing, Inc.
All rights reserved. This book or any portion thereof may not be reproduced or used in any manner whatsoever without the express written permission of the publisher except for the use of brief quotations in a book review.

Julia Grady

First edition: 2014

Disclaimer/Limit of Liability

This book is for informational purposes only. The views expressed are those of the author alone, and should not be taken as expert, legal, or medical advice. The reader is responsible for his or her own actions.

Every attempt has been made to verify the accuracy of the information in this publication. However, neither the author nor the publisher assumes any responsibility for errors, omissions, or contrary interpretation of the material contained herein.

This book is not intended to provide medical advice. Please see your health care professional before embarking on any new diet or exercise program. The reader should regularly consult a physician in matters relating to his/her health and particularly with respect to any symptoms that may require diagnosis or medical attention.

Contents

Introduction 1

Essential Oils Basics 3
    What Are Essential Oils? 3
    History of Aromatherapy and 4
    Essential Oils 4
    Science of Aromatherapy 5
    Benefits and Uses of Essential Oils and Aromatherapy 7

Buying and Storing 11

Essential Oils 11
    Extraction Processes 11
    Quality of Essential Oils 17
    Buying Essential Oils 17
    Storing Your Oils 19

Using Essential Oils 21
    Safety Considerations 21
    Proper Dilution of Essential Oils 23
    Carrier Oils 25
    Application Methods 26

Creating Your Own 31

Essential Oil Blends 31

Aromatic Blending vs. Therapeutic Blending *31*
Blending 101 .... *32*
Basic Rules for Blending *33*
Essential Oil Notes *35*
The Order of Blending *36*
Creating Your Blend *37*
Tools and Supplies *38*

Essential Oils A to Z 41

Allspice 43
Amyris 45
Angelica 46
Anise Seed 47
Balsam Fir 48
Basil 49
Bay Laurel 50
Bay West Indies 51
Benzoin 52
Bergamot 54
Black Pepper 56
Blue Cyprus 58
Blue Tansy 60
Cajeput 61
Camphor 63
Cardamom 64
Carrot Seed 66
Catnip 67
Cedarwood 68
Celery Seed 69
Chamomile, German 70
Chamomile, Roman 72
Cilantro 74
Cinnamon (leaf) 75
Cistus 77
Citronella 78
Clary Sage 79
Clove 81

Combava Petitgrain	83
Copaiba	84
Coriander	85
Cornmint	86
Cypress	87
Davana	89
Dill Seed	90
Dorado Azul	91
Douglas Fir	92
Elemi	93
Eucalyptus	94
Fennel	95
Fir Needle	97
Frankincense	98
Galbanum	100
Geranium	101
Ginger	103
Goldenrod	105
Grapefruit	106
Helichrysum	108
Hinoki	110
Hops	111
Ho Wood	112
Hyssop	113
Idaho Blue Spruce	114
Jasmine	115
Juniper	117
Lavandin	118
Lavender	119
Ledum	121
Lemon	122
Lemon Balm (Melissa)	124
Lemon Myrtle	125
Lemongrass	126
Lime	128
Litsea Cubeba	129
Lovage Leaf	130
Mace	131
Mandarin	132
Manuka	133

Marjoram	135
Mountain Savory	136
Myrrh	137
Myrtle	139
Neroli	140
Niaouli	142
Nutmeg	143
Oak Moss	145
Orange, Bitter	146
Orange, Sweet	147
Oregano	149
Palmarosa	151
Palo Santo	152
Parsley Seed	153
Patchouli	154
Pennyroyal	156
Peppermint	157
Peru Balsam	159
Petitgrain	160
Pine (Scotch Pine)	161
Ravensara	162
Rose	163
Rosemary	165
Sage	167
Sandalwood	168
Spearmint	170
Spikenard	172
Spruce, Black	173
Spruce (Hemlock or Eastern)	174
St. John's Wort	175
Tagetes	176
Tangerine	177
Tansy, Idaho	178
Tarragon	179
Tea Tree	180
Thyme	182
Tumeric	184
Valerian	185
Vanilla	186
Vetiver	188
Wintergreen	190

Yarrow 191
  Ylang Ylang 193

Recipes 195
  Mood Enhancement 195
  Stress Relief 204
  Headaches 207
  Colds and Flu 209
  Insomnia and Sleep Disorders 211
  Skin and Hair Care 212
  Home and Yard 219
  Pets 222

Index of Symptoms 225

Conclusion 237

Resources and 239

References 239
  Books on Essential Oils and 239
  Aromatherapy 239
  Sources of Essential Oils 240

From the Author 244

Introduction

Interest in essential oils and aromatherapy is on the rise, and with good reason. Aromatherapy is a method that uses the sense of smell to influence the brain and body to relieve pain and stress, boost mood, increase energy, fight fatigue, decrease appetite, lose weight, and a host of other purposes. Each essential oil has its own unique properties and produces different results. For example, eucalyptus may be used as a pick-me-up after a long day, while lavender will help you relax and fall asleep.

The sense of smell is very powerful. It can influence our emotions and trigger memories. Smells travel by way of the olfactory nerves up to the area of the brain called the limbic system. This area of the brain is responsible for our moods, feelings, and memory, as well as conditioned responses and learning. When the limbic system is stimulated, it releases neurotransmitters, endorphins, and other "feel-good" chemicals. In this way, aromatherapy and essential oils can alter the brain's chemistry.

Essential oils also work by being absorbed through the skin into the blood stream. They can be added to carrier oils, lotions, creams, and other ointments and massaged into the skin to relieve tired muscles, aches and pains, as well as a variety of skin conditions. Used in this way, they are safe and effective natural remedies.

Essential oils have been used for thousands of years and have been shown to be beneficial for a variety of purposes. These all-natural oils are an excellent alternative and complementary approach to improving health, and when used properly, have very few side effects. As people rediscover the many benefits that can be obtained from using essential oils, they will continue to increase in use and popularity.

This book is designed to be a complete guide to understanding and using essential oils. Part I starts with a history of essential oils, their benefits and uses, along with safety tips and precautions. We then turn to how to use essential oils, buying and storing advice, carrier oils, application methods, as well as tools and techniques for blending. Part II is an A-to-Z resource of all the major (and some minor, lesser known) essential oils. It takes a comprehensive look at each oil's characteristics, properties, therapeutic uses, and suggested blends. Part III includes a variety of recipes for everything from anxiety and depression to weight loss, pet care, and household cleaners. Also included is an index of symptoms and ailments to make it easy to find the correct essential oil for your specific needs.

Read on to discover all of the many benefits that aromatherapy and essential oils have in store for you and your family.

Essential Oils Basics

What Are Essential Oils?

They are the natural oils that are extracted from plants, including from the leaves, stem, flowers, fruits, bark, and even roots. Do not confuse them with perfumes, which are fabricated substances without healing properties. Unlike perfumes, essential oils do not contain any synthetic ingredients and they have known benefits for both the mind and body.

Essential oils contain various chemical components that influence the different systems in the body. This may sound somewhat dangerous, but it actually isn't because our bodies naturally produce and use many of these same chemical compounds already. The essential oils work by stimulating or sedating the body's systems. Many also contain powerful anti-inflammatory, antiviral, antibacterial, antifungal, and other properties.

For example, ester, a chemical component found in bergamot, chamomile, lavender, and sage, acts as a sedative, a calming agent, an antifungal, and an anti-inflammatory. Ketones, substances that promote new cell growth and help wounds heal faster, are found in camphor, eucalyptus, rosemary, and sage. Alcohols, which act as diuretics and fight bacteria, are contained in ginger, patchouli, peppermint, rose, rosewood, sandalwood, and tea tree, as well as other essential oils.

History of Aromatherapy and Essential Oils

In science there is a concept known as quintessence. It is a force that is ever present, but hard to define. In the past 20 years, this concept became popular in physics and has been discussed as a dark energy. Although how it works is still unclear, it represents the idea of an indefinable dynamic energy that exists in our universe.

The idea of this unknown force is not new. Long ago, Aristotle proposed the existence of a fifth element (in addition to fire, water, air, and earth) that existed in nature. He described the fifth element as a life force, or spirit. It was later known as an essential element.

While the term quintessence is unfamiliar to most people, the idea of an essential element is not. Many years ago, philosophers continued to test Aristotle's theory of quintessence. The result of their research led to the development of a product we recognize today as essential oils.

Essential oils and aromatherapy have been used for thousands of years for therapeutic as well as spiritual purposes. Their use dates back to the ancient civilizations of Egypt, Greece, Rome, and China.

Essential oils were used as incense and burned as part of religious rituals by the Egyptians, as well as in the mummification process. They were also widely used in cosmetics and perfumes and for healing purposes.

Ancient healers, including Hippocrates, recognized the healing powers contained in many plants and natural remedies were discovered and used effectively to treat and cure a variety of ailments.

However, during the Middle Ages, much of the knowledge and interest in the science of aromatherapy was lost, mostly due to the influence of the Catholic Church. Some cultures kept it alive though, such as the Chinese, where essential oils have long been a part of traditional Chinese medicine.

The healing power of plants was rediscovered, quite by accident, by the French chemist René-Maurice Gattefossé, who, while working in his laboratory in the 1920s, accidently burned his hand. He applied lavender oil to it, and was amazed at the healing effect it had on his burns. This led him to further study the properties of many essential oils and eventually the founding of modern-day aromatherapy.

It has only been in the last few decades that interest in alternative and natural medicine has made a comeback. This interest has inspired many to turn to aromatherapy and essential oils and rediscover their many amazing uses and benefits.

Science of Aromatherapy

Aromatherapy is the practice of using the essences derived from beneficial plants to heal the body. It is also known as essential oil therapy because the aromatic essence is obtained from essential oils. The oils may be inhaled, applied topically, and in some cases ingested.

Aromatherapy is based on the use of plants to balance and harmonize the psychological, spiritual, and physical aspects of the human body. Once this balance is achieved, the body can better heal itself.

When an essential oil is inhaled its scent is carried through the nose to the brain via olfactory nerve cells. Upon reaching the brain, the scent activates the limbic center, which is the part of the brain responsible for emotions, among other functions. Neurotransmitters such as serotonin and dopamine, as well as endorphins, are released. Depending upon the essential oil inhaled, you may feel aroused, excited, or more relaxed.

Although the name places emphasis on the aromatic essence of plants, aromatherapy is not just about smells. The oils used in aromatherapy are rich in antioxidants and work to combat free radicals throughout the body. Their antioxidant power is much stronger than those found in the fruits and vegetables that are typically eaten. In addition, they have the ability to react with hormones and enzymes in the body causing noticeable reactions. When using aromatherapy it is not uncommon to see changes in pulse or blood pressure. Certain oils also stimulate the body's natural ability to ignore pain.

Benefits and Uses of Essential Oils and Aromatherapy

Aromatherapy is commonly used to promote general relaxation, increase feelings of well-being, and reduce stress. While aromatherapy is very effective for altering mood, essential oils can have positive effects on many other levels. They are also used to boost the immune system and fight inflammation throughout the body. In addition, they can be used to treat infections, relieve pain, and promote healing.

There are hundreds of different essential oils, many of which are only occasionally used and some of which are known poisons. There also a multitude of known uses. Here we list some of the most common uses of essential oils.

Mood Enhancement

One thing many essential oils are used for is the regulation of mood. Ranging from the ability to arouse to the ability relax, essential oils can lead to a wide variety of changes in how you perceive your environment.

Muscle Relaxation

Essential oils are frequently used in massage oils and lotions, making them particularly useful for treating muscle discomfort. They can be used to reduce muscle spasms, promote healing, and aid in overall relaxation. When combined with massage they are a powerful form of therapy.

Skincare

The antibacterial, anti-inflammatory, and antiseptic properties of many essential oils make them an ideal addition for skincare products. When added to cosmetics, balms, or lotions, certain oils can help prevent scars, combat acne, heal dry skin, reduce the appearance of stretch marks, ease rashes, and promote wound healing.

Pain Relief

Essential oils can also be a powerful source of pain relief. Many are natural analgesics, containing substances such as methyl salicylate the main ingredient in aspirin, and when used can block the body's pain receptors. Wintergreen oil contains a high concentration of methyl salicylate and it has been documented that this oil can have cortisone-like effects that can get to the root of pain and provide fast relief. Wintergreen has been used for centuries as an effective pain reliever.

Anti-Inflammation

Chronic inflammation is thought to be the root cause of many diseases today including heart disease, cancer, diabetes, and arthritis. Research has shown essential oils to have the ability to reduce inflammation.

COX enzymes are responsible for the body's inflammatory response. Several essential oils work as proven COX inhibitors, reducing inflammation throughout the body. These oils are thyme, clove, cinnamon, fennel, eucalyptus, bergamot, and rose.

In addition, many essential oils can improve blood flow and circulation by reducing the amount of nitric oxide in the body. Nitric oxide has been linked to the type of inflammation attributed to high blood pressure, heart disease, and diabetes.

Weight Loss

Essential oils are effective at promoting weight loss. They do this by suppressing appetite, boosting metabolism and increasing the rate at which the body burns fat, curbing sugar and carb cravings, reducing bloating and water retention, and general detoxification. By regulating emotions, they can also reduce overeating linked to stress and other emotional issues.

Multi Purpose

The properties of essential oils are complex and work together in a synergistic fashion on multiple systems. This is why just one essential oil can be used for so many different symptoms. When used in combination, their power increases exponentially.

Essential Oils for Beginners

Buying and Storing Essential Oils

Extraction Processes

While it is true that essential oils are an essential part of aromatherapy, the term essential doesn't mean essential as in "being a necessary part of." Instead, essential oils are the oils extracted from the essence of a plant, that is, those parts that contain the plant's aroma molecules.

Using different methods of extraction guarantees that the highest concentration of oils can be obtained. Many different parts of plants are used to extract essential oils from—flowers, fruits, herbs, stems, roots, leaves, buds, blossoms, seeds, nuts, and even tree bark produce some of the most aromatic and therapeutic essential oils. Essential oil extraction methods fall under three main categories: distillation, expression, and solvent extraction. The following is an overview of these extraction processes and methods.

Steam Distillation
Most essential oils are extracted using a steam distillation process. It is the oldest form of essential oil extraction and

some believe it to be the only way oils should be extracted. The process really is pretty simple and as long as the extraction process is closely monitored, the steam will remain at a temperature that won't damage the plants.

In steam distillation, the plant material is placed onto a still, which is a specialized piece of equipment that is used in the distillation process. It consists of a container into which heat is added and an apparatus that is used for cooling. The plant is first placed into the container and then steam is added and passed through the plant. The heat from the steam helps to open the parts of the plant that contain the plant's aromatic molecules or oils. Once open, the plant releases these aromatic molecules and they are able to rise along with the steam.

The vapors carrying these molecules travel in a closed system toward the cooling apparatus. Cold water is then used to cool the vapors. As they cool, they condense and transform into a liquid state. The liquid is collected into a container and, as with any type of oil and water mixture, it separates. The oils float to the top while the water settles at the bottom. From there, it's a simple matter of removing the oils that have been separated. These are the highly condensed, aromatic oils used in aromatherapy.

However, the water is not simply discarded. This water also contains the plant's aroma, along with the other parts of the plant that are water soluble. These are known as hydrosols. They are milder than essential oils and are also used in aromatherapy.

Water Distillation

Another type of distillation is water distillation, which involves placing the desired plant material into a still and then submerging it in water. Then, the water is brought to a boil. The heat helps open the parts of the plant that contain the plant's aromatic molecules so they can be extracted. The vapors cool and condense, the essential oils separate from the water, and they're collected.

The water provides protection for the plant during this process because it acts as a barrier. In addition, less pressure and a lower temperature are used than that which is used in steam distillation. This type of extraction method works well with plants that cannot tolerate high heat.

Expression

Essential oil extraction via expression does not involve the use of a heat. This is the method commonly used to extract oils from the rinds of citrus. In earlier times, rinds were squeezed by hand and a sponge was used to collect the essential oils. The fruit would be removed and then the rinds, along with the pith, would be soaked in water to make them easier to work with. Then, they would be turned upside-down which caused the cells containing the oils to break apart. Once broken, the oils would drip out and soak into a nearby sponge. When the sponge became saturated, the oils were squeezed into a container so they could be decanted.

Ecuelle a Picuer

Another expression method involved sticking pins into the skins of fruit for the purpose of damaging the cells that contain the essential oils. The apparatus used had a built-in container for collecting the oils and the other parts of the fruit that ended up in the collection area. The final steps involved separating the essential oils and decanting them. This is called the *ecuelle a picuer* method.

Machine Abrasion

Those were quite labor-intensive processes, and thankfully, technological advances led to the invention of machines to do this type of tedious work. Nowadays, oils from rinds are extracted using centrifugal force. This rapid process is called machine abrasion.

Cold Pressed

This form of expression extraction is also used to extract essential oils from nuts and seeds and from the rinds of citrus. Mechanical pressure is used to force the oils out. The oils extracted contain water, but this water will, in time, evaporate, leaving just the essential oils. The downside of using this extraction method is that the cold pressed oils spoil more quickly than those extracted using other methods. That's why it's important to purchase these types of essential oils in small quantities so you don't have to end up throwing them out.

Solvent Extraction

Some plant material cannot tolerate the high heats used in other extraction methods such as steam distillation. The heat damages these plants, and once damaged their essential oils are also spoiled and no longer able to be used. In these cases, solvents such as alcohol, ether, ethanol, methanol, hexane, and even petroleum are used instead.

The problem with using solvents to extract essential oils is that most of the time, residual solvents or impurities remain in the end product. Because of these impurities, some aromatherapists do not use them.

However, there are times when solvent extraction makes sense. In this process, the plant material is first washed in a bath of hydrocarbon solvents. This dissolves the necessary plant materials including the aromatic molecules, waxy matter, and pigment, and the dissolved matter mixes in with the solvent. The solvent mixture is then filtered and distilled using low pressure. After distillation and further processing, either a resin or a concentrate remains. Additional processing using alcohol helps extract the essential oils.

This type of extraction is very fast and cost-effective, but there is a downside. With solvent extraction, residual solvents remain and their presence can cause problems if used by individuals with allergies or sensitive skin. That's another reason why essential oils extracted using solvents are typically used in the manufacturing of perfumes and fragrances, and not in aromatherapy or skin care products.

Maceration

In this extraction method, hot oil is used as a way to rip apart cell membranes. The plant material is first saturated with hot oil and then allowed to soak until the cell membranes rupture. As they break apart, essential oils are released into the oil in which the plant material is soaking. The plant material is then removed from the oil and the oil that remains gets decanted.

Carbon Dioxide (CO2) Extraction

One of the newest extraction technologies uses carbon dioxide. The end result of carbon dioxide (CO_2) extraction is a super-concentrated, high-quality version of the essential oil. This rapid extraction method uses lower temperatures and higher pressure to transform carbon dioxide, a gas, into a liquid. It's an inert solvent, meaning that it's non-reactive and therefore cannot form another chemical compound. When the extraction process is complete, the carbon dioxide is returned back to a gaseous state and no residual remains. All that is left is pure essential oil.

Although this technology produces one of the purest forms of essential oil, it is not yet widely used. This is because the equipment needed for this extraction process is very expensive, which keeps production costs high. Also, because production costs are high, so too are the costs of the essential oils that are produced this way.

Quality of Essential Oils

The quality of essential oils is highly variable and as a consumer it can be difficult to determine if you are purchasing a high-quality oil. Essential oils are regulated by the Food and Drug Administration (FDA) and they are classified either as cosmetics, food, or drugs, depending upon their intended use. How the FDA classifies them varies, but most are not considered drugs by the FDA and are instead considered cosmetics or fragrances.

Many factors go into the production of essential oils and things like soil quality, growing conditions, and harvesting methods can all make a difference in the final product. In addition, some companies selling essential oils will dilute or adulterate the oil in some way and this can be hard to identify. It is important to find pure, unadulterated oils because otherwise the oil will not be as potent and may not have the intended effects.

The grade of the essential oil is another factor to consider. While essential oils are not actually "graded" by an outside regulatory body, many essential oils are sold in different grades and these can be a good indicator of quality. The higher graded oils are typically purer, single-sourced, and higher quality and, of course, command higher prices.

Buying Essential Oils

Once you enter into the world of aromatherapy, you'll soon realize that along with the many enticing scents, there is also a multitude of purchasing sources. It can be confusing to decide where to purchase your essential oils. The following are some issues to consider.

Make sure you read the labels and the product descriptions. Know what you are purchasing, whether online or offline. Look for labels containing the words "pure" or "100 percent" essential oil. Anything else, and the product is most likely diluted with either a carrier oil or other additives, and you will not be getting a true essential oil. Also, some companies may be trying to pass off synthetic oils as true essential oils.

In addition, know your prices before you shop. By knowing which oils you would expect to pay more for, such as those considered rare or exotic, you'll have a better idea whether or not the asking price is accurate. The price of aromatherapy products and ingredients will vary but still should fall within some commonly accepted price ranges.

Steer clear from essential oils that are bottled using clear or plastic bottles. Light and plastic can damage and contaminate these oils. Dark-colored glass bottles—amber or dark blue—are best for storage.

Also, watch out for dust. Why? An essential oil's properties, and therefore its effectiveness, will start to diminish over time. Dust is a sign that the bottle's already spent some time on the shelf and perhaps isn't as fresh as it could be. Of course, if you're purchasing online you won't be able to see this factor.

Once you have found a source for essential oils that you're comfortable with, it's wise to become a loyal customer. Since essential oils are all-natural, consistency can be a challenge. You might find a single source offers you the best chance of getting a consistent high-quality product.

Check out the resources section at the back of the book for a list of sources for high-quality essential oils.

Storing Your Oils

How you store your oils will have a big impact on their shelf life. Left under the wrong conditions, these delicate oils can break down and become worthless.

First, be sure your oils are kept in dark-colored glass bottles. This will protect them from harmful ultraviolet light. This is most likely how you purchased them, but if for some reason they were purchased in clear or plastic bottles then be sure to transfer them as soon as possible.

Next, remember that essential oils do not like extremes of heat or light. Do no place them out on a window shelf in the sun, regardless of how pretty they may look decorating your window! This will cause them to deteriorate very quickly. So find a cool dark place and keep them there. Some people keep their essential oils in the refrigerator, especially citrus oils which like it cool. Just make sure they don't get confused with your edible items. Be sure to take them out of the refrigerator a couple of hours before using them to allow any fatty particles to re-dissolve. Give them a shake before using to make sure all of the particles are dissolved evenly.

Remember to place the caps back tightly on the bottles when you have finished with them. Otherwise, the essential oils will evaporate.

Proper storage of essential oils is also a significant concern for safety reasons. Some essential oils are toxins if ingested and they are also flammable. The smells may be very enticing to someone, such as a child, who does not know what they are and they may attempt to eat them. This can have disastrous results. In terms of flammability, the distillation process makes it very similar to alcohol, and highly sensitive to open flames. For these reasons, be sure to store the oils out of reach of children.

Using Essential Oils

Safety Considerations

Although essential oils are natural products that have been used for thousands of years, there are certain safety precautions to keep in mind.

First, the majority of essential oils are meant to be inhaled or applied topically. They are not meant to be ingested and can be toxic or even fatal if consumed.

Many essential oils can irritate the skin and mucous membranes. Pure undiluted oil should not be used directly on the skin. They are extremely powerful in this form and may cause an adverse reaction.

As a general rule, essential oil therapy should not be used in pregnancy, by lactating women, or young children. There are some exceptions to this rule but it is a good idea to check with your health practitioner before using any essential oil in these situations.

Keep all essential oils out of reach of children. Remember to treat essential oils as the medicines that they are. While they may smell good, they are extremely powerful and are never safe for children to ingest.

If you are suffering from any chronic health condition or take prescription medications then please check with your health practitioner before embarking on essential oil therapy to avoid possible contraindications. People with asthma, epilepsy, kidney or liver conditions should be especially careful when using essential oils.

Patch Test

Some essential oils can cause an allergic reaction or sensitization in some individuals.

Before using any essential oil it is important to do a patch test on a small area of skin to check for any type of allergic or other type of adverse reaction. Apply a small amount of diluted oil to your inner arm. Wait 24 hours to check for redness or irritation to develop. If it does, wash the area with soap and water and do not use the oil.

Phototoxicity

Sun sensitivity, otherwise known as phototoxicity, can occur when using certain essential oils. What this means is that your skin will be more sensitive to sunlight and more prone to sunburn in the period following use of the oil. The following oils have been known to induce phototoxicity and should not be applied to skin that will be in direct sunlight within 24 hours: angelica, bergamot, citrus oils, cumin, dill, tagetes, yuzu.

Ingestion of Essential Oils

As stated previously, it is not recommended that essential oils should ever be ingested. Do so only under the guidance of a qualified professional.

In case of accidental ingestion, call your local poison control center.

Hazardous Oils

Certain essential oils should not be used in home aromatherapy preparations. These include wormwood, pennyroyal, camphor, wintergreen, and bitter almond. Use of these essential oils should only be used with the guidance of a qualified professional.

Proper Dilution of Essential Oils

As mentioned previously, it is almost never a good idea to apply essential oils to the skin undiluted, or "neat." Although it is sometimes said that certain oils such as lavender or tea tree oil may be safely applied this way, even these oils have been know to cause sensitization reactions. It is not necessary to use essential oils undiluted in order to gain their therapeutic properties and it is not worth the risk.

Always dilute your essential oils in a carrier oil (see next section on carrier oils) before application. Simply place the desired number of drops of essential oil into the carrier oil and mix. Below is a quick-reference guide for making common dilution strengths.

> ***1 percent dilution:** *6 drops per 1 ounce (30 ml) of carrier oil.* This strength is recommended for people with sensitive skin, health conditions, children, and pregnant women. Also for massaging over large areas.

> ***2 percent dilution:*** *12 drops per 1 ounce (30 ml) of carrier oil.* This is the standard dilution for most people and is the one recommended for most purposes.
>
> ***5 percent dilution:*** *30 drops per 1 ounce (30 ml) of carrier oil.* Use this strength short term for a particular condition such as congestion or muscle pain.
>
> ***10 percent dilution:*** *60 drops per 1 ounce (30 ml) of carrier oil.* Use for temporary relief of specific conditions.
>
> ***25 percent dilution:*** *150 drops per 1 ounce (30 ml) of carrier oil.* This strength would be used occasionally for situations such as severe pain, cramping, or bruising.

Here is another quick reference guide for making conversions to smaller amounts. These are all amounts for making a 2 percent dilution.

> **Essential Oil : Carrier Oil (2% dilution)**
>
> 2 drops : 5 ml
>
> 4 drops : 10 ml
>
> 6 drops : 15 ml
>
> 8 drops : 20 ml
>
> 12 drops : 30 ml
>
> 20 drops : 50 ml
>
> 40 drops : 100 ml

Carrier Oils

Carrier oils are an important part of aromatherapy and there are quite a few to choose from. Vegetable and nut oils make the most effective carrier oils. But remember, do not simply reach into your kitchen cabinet and pull out a vegetable oil that you use for cooking. Why? Because oils used for cooking go through a different manufacturing process than the carrier oils that are used in aromatherapy. These processes are harsh and they actually strip out much of the vegetable oil's useful vitamins, nutrients, and fatty acids.

When shopping for carrier oils to use in aromatherapy, look for oils that have been cold-pressed. This is a natural process and it does not involve chemicals or heat, which ensures that the beneficial fatty acids and other nutrients are retained within the oil.

Also, be sure to select carrier oils that have little or no odor. You don't want the oil's scent to compete with your essential oil. A carrier oil should be light and not have a sticky feel. These qualities ensure the oils will penetrate easily and efficiently.

There are many different types of carrier oils suitable for aromatherapy. Sunflower oil, coconut oil, avocado oil, olive oil, jojoba oil, evening primrose oil, sweet almond oil, grapeseed oil, macadamia oil, and wheat germ oil are all good choices. Since each will have different qualities such as aroma, texture, and color, selecting the right one is a matter of personal preference. Carrier oils will also interact differently depending on the essential oil with which it's mixed.

A type of carrier oil to avoid is mineral oil. Both mineral oil and petroleum jelly are the byproducts of petrochemical processing. Mineral oil is commonly used in baby oil and other moisturizers because it is an inexpensive oil. However, it is not a natural product and should not be used in aromatherapy. It can prevent the essential oils from being properly absorbed and contains toxins that may be absorbed through the skin into the body. The same applies to petroleum jelly.

Application Methods

Once your essential oil has been mixed, it is ready to be used. Essential oil blends can be used in a variety of manners by adding the created blend to other items. Popular uses include spraying as a mist, massage oils, skincare products, homeopathic medicine, as well as cleaning supplies. Essential oil blends allow you to create custom scents and therapies for your situation.

Topical Application

Applying diluted essential oils directly to the skin is one of the most popular and effective application methods.

Massage

Massaging essential oils into the skin is a commonly used aromatherapy technique and one that'll enable you to reap tremendous therapeutic benefits. Simply mix with your chosen carrier oil. As a general rule, you'll need 1 to 2 ounces of carrier oil to massage the entire body.

Creams and Lotions

You can also purchase unscented facial creams and body lotions and then add your own essential oils to them.

Bath

Adding essential oils to your bath water is a wonderful way to reap their benefits. Simply add 5-10 drops to the water.

Compress

Using a warm or cold compress that has been soaked in essential oils is an effective method for relieving certain skin conditions, bruises, and wounds, as well as muscular aches and pains. Add 5-10 drops to 6 ounces of water, soak cloth, and apply.

Inhalation

Steam inhalation of essential oils are useful for relieving congestion as well as treating colds, flus, and sinus infections. Place 5-10 drops of essentia oil into a large bowl of boiling water. Cover your head with a towel and breathe in through your nose. Keep your eyes closed to avoid irritation.

You can also apply a couple of drops of essential oil to a cotton ball or handkerchief and then inhale the scent.

Diffusion

There are many ways aromatherapy oils can be diffused including several methods that make use of items you likely have lying around the house.

A **lamp ring** fits on a light bulb. This popular option is made using terra cotta. The lamp ring has a groove into which essential oils are placed. When the lamp is turned on, the heat from the bulb heats the ring, which in turn heats the oils. As oils are heated, they get diffused into the atmosphere.

Clay pots, also made from terra cotta, are another type of inexpensive commercial solution. With these, essential oils aren't heated, they're simply poured into and stored within the pot. To activate, you remove the cork and the aroma from the oils is released.

A **candle diffuser** is a self-contained unit that utilizes a small candle as a heat source and a tray for holding oils. When the candle is lit, the heat from the flame warms the oils, which then release their aromas. There are many styles of candle diffuser available.

Fan diffusers don't use heat and are more efficient at disbursing aromas than the previous types of diffusers. Essential oils are placed onto an absorbent pad that is then inserted into the appropriate fan opening. Cool air blows over the pad, picks up the scent and carries it throughout the room. Fan diffusers can be electric or battery operated. Make sure to use a fan that is large enough to accommodate the room size.

An **electric heat diffuser** is a unit that first heats the oil and then uses a built-in fan to diffuse them.

The most sophisticated (and expensive) aromatherapy diffusion product is the **nebulizer**. This three-part system consists of an electric pump, a glass container, and a tubing/cork. The pump forces small amounts of essential oils through the twisted glass. This action breaks the oils into tiny droplets that are then dispersed throughout the room.

Ingestion

As previously mentioned, it is not recommended that essential oils are ingested. This should be done only under the guidance of a qualified professional.

Essential Oils for Beginners

Creating Your Own Essential Oil Blends

As you get more involved in aromatherapy, there will probably come a time when you will want to start experimenting with making your own blends. Blending is simply the combining of different essential oils and carrier oils for the purpose of achieving different results.

Once you understand the theory behind blending, it's something you'll easily be able to do on your own. However, if you'd prefer not to, there are plenty of sources of premade aromatherapy blends.

Aromatic Blending vs. Therapeutic Blending

The difference between the two main types of aromatherapy blending is pretty straightforward. The goal in aromatic blending is to make a great smelling blend. The goal in therapeutic blending is to create a mixture that will alleviate a certain symptom or condition, such as body aches or pain or stress reduction. Although the scent is not the focus with therapeutic blending it is still an important factor to consider. If the blend smells horrible, you may not want to use it!

Blending 101

Not all combinations of oils will complement one another. This is probably one of the most important things you need to keep in mind before you begin aromatherapy blending. Sometimes the properties of one essential oil will overwhelm the others, and therefore they should not be mixed together, or only small amounts should be added into a blend. You don't have to spend countless time experimenting yourself to learn which essential oil properties work well together and which don't. We've given a list of suggested blends that work together with each oil in the A-to-Z guide.

When blending, it's better to limit the number of oils you combine to three, sometimes four, until you're more experienced with the process.

To blend the oils, the jar containing the essential oils should be rolled between the palms of your two hands. No need to shake it up.

Another thing to keep in mind is documenting your blend recipe. When you create a fantastic blend, you'll want to be able recall the ingredients as well as the proportions you used. Likewise, when creating a blend that just doesn't work or causes irritation, you'll know what *not* to do next time.

When composing blends, contraindications, or any factors that would prohibit use of a certain ingredient, must be identified and avoided. For example, there are a number of different oils that should be avoided during pregnancy. Allergic reactions are another contraindication to be keep in mind. If you are allergic to something, such as nuts, then nut oils should definitely be avoided in your blends. Contraindications are a matter of personal safety and should be taken seriously.

Finally, for safety reasons as well as for organization, always properly label and store your aromatherapy blends as well as the individual ingredients in a cool, dark area away from pets and children.

Basic Rules for Blending

Essential oil blending has a few basic principles to consider when combining all types of oils. The first thing to consider is the oil's chemical properties. Aspects of the oil such as its viscosity (thickness) and volatility (how reactive it is) should always be considered before blending. Otherwise, one of the oils may completely overpower the other oil, resulting in an ineffective blend.

Another aspect to consider is the desired effects of the blend. Oils that are complementary should be blended together. It wouldn't make much sense to blend an essential oil that has energizing properties with one that has calming properties if your intent was to invigorate.

The final, and perhaps most overlooked aspect of blending to consider is the order of blending. Believe it or not, the oils must be added in a certain order in order to achieve the desired effect. This is because of the chemical properties of the oils. An essential oil that has stronger properties may need to be diluted by certain other essential oils in order to receive a desired effect. However, the same oil might dilute other oils in different mixtures. Because of the vast possibility of mixtures, it is important to thoroughly understand the different properties of the oils you are working with before you start blending.

Below is a helpful chart which organizes some common essential oils by aroma types.

Aroma Category

Camphorous/Medicinal: Cajuput, Eucalyptus, Tea Tree

Citrus: Lemon, Lime, Orange, Tangerine

Earthy: Oakmoss, Vetiver, Patchouli

Floral: Jasmine, Lavender, Neroli, Rose

Herbaceous: Basil, Marjoram, Rosemary

Minty: Peppermint, Spearmint

Oriental: Ginger, Patchouli

Spicy: Clove, Cinnamon, Nutmeg

Woodsy: Cedar, Pine

In general, essential oils in the same category blend well with one another. In addition, here are a few general guidelines for what works well together:

- Florals blend well with citrusy, spicy, and woodsy scents.
- Minty scents blend well with citrus, earthy, herbaceous, and woodsy scents.
- Oriental scents blend well with citrus, florals, and spicy scents.
- Spicy scents blend well with citrus, florals, and orientals.
- Woodsy oils blend well with most other scents.

Essential Oil Notes

Although there are a wide variety of essential oils, they have been classified into three groups for blending purposes. These groups are called *notes*, and they are based on the chemical properties of the oils.

Essential oils that are made of small and light molecules are called top notes. These oils are thin, absorb quickly into the skin, and evaporate quickly. These oils tend to be light, fresh, and uplifting.

Middle notes make up the majority of essential oils. These oils usually do not have a very strong scent and are used to give body to the blend and balance it out.

Base notes usually have a heavy scent and evaporate the slowest. These essential oils have a rich, deep scent, and tend to be the most expensive oils.

The best blend would include combinations from each of these notes.

Below is a chart with the note classifications of common essential oils.

> **Top Notes**
>
> Anise, Basil, Bay Laurel, Bergamont, Citronella, Eucalyptus, Galbanum, Grapefruit, Lavender, Lavendin, Lemon, Lemongrass, Lime, Orange, Peppermint, Petitgrain, Spearmint, Tagetes, Tangerine
>
> **Middle Notes**
>
> Bat, Cajeput, Carrot Seed, Chamomile (German and Roman), Cinnamon, Clary Sage, Clove, Cypress, Dill, Elemi, Fennel, Fir, Geranium, Hyssop, Jasmine, Juniper Berry, Linden, Marjoram, Neroli, Nutmeg, Palmarosa, Parsley, Pepper, Pine, Rose, Rosemary, Rosewood, Spruce, Tea Tree, Thyme, Yarrow, Ylang Ylang
>
> **Base Notes**
>
> Angelica Root, Balsam, Benzoin, Cedarwood, Frankincense, Ginger, Helichrysum, Myrrh, Oakmoss, Olibanum, Patchouli, Sandalwood, Vanilla, Vetiver

The Order of Blending

As mentioned earlier, the order in which blends are created makes a huge difference in how an essential oil blend will perform. To help simplify the process, essential oils can be separated into four function categories.

Every essential oil blend starts with the oil that will determine the personality of the blend. This oil is typically long lasting with a strong aroma. Because this oil is so strong, it should only make up 1-5 percent of the total essential oil mixture. It is called the *personifier* because a large majority of the therapeutic action of the blend will come from it.

The second oil that is added to an essential oil blend is designed to enhance the effects of the first oil. These *enhancers* tend to have a strong aroma and can make up 50-80 percent of the blend. These are the oils you will most likely recognize in the final blend.

The third group of essential oils are the *equalizers*. These oils balance the other oils and help optimize the therapeutic effects. Their effects do not last as long as the other oils, and do not have a strong aroma. They can be anywhere from 10-50 percent of the blend.

If a fourth group of essential oils is used in your blend, it will most likely be a *modifier*. These oils do not have a strong aroma and they do not last very long. Like the equalizer, they are added to improve the collaboration of the other oils. Modifiers can make up 5-8 percent of an essential oil blend.

Creating Your Blend

The ratio for essential oil to carrier oils will be determined by your desired use. For therapeutic usage, some practitioners will create blends that are up to 10 percent essential oil. This means that 90 percent of the oil is made up of carrier oil.

To understand percentages for blending it is best to mix your blends in terms of ounces. This is preferable for a couple of reasons. One reason is because by using a standard 1 ounce system you are better able to control the amount of essential oil you add to each blend, and guarantee a standard result. Another reason why you would want to create blends in 1 ounce increments is because essential oil blends do not last long. By creating only as much as you immediately need, you do not have to worry about it losing its potency over time.

It is typically recommended that home essential oil blends be made to a 1-2 percent dilution. One percent is appropriate for those who may have adverse affects to the blends (such as children or pregnant women), 2 percent is strong enough for most people. Oils for massage therapy are typically created to be 2 percent. Mixtures of 3 percent and greater are very powerful and should be reserved for short-term use for a specific purpose or with the guidance of an experienced practitioner.

See the section on Proper Dilution of Essential Oils for a chart on dilution ratios.

Tools and Supplies

In order to create an essential oil blend you will need a few basic supplies.

*Glass droppers. These allow small measurements of the essential oil into the carrier oil. They will also ensure that you do not put too much essential oil in the blend.

***Rods.** Glass rods for mixing are your best bet since these will be nonreactive with the oils.

***Glass containers.** Blends should be stored in dark colored glass containers, preferably 4 ounces and smaller. Do not fill to the top, the blend needs room to breathe. Add half of the carrier oil to the container, then the essential oils, then finally the remainder of the carrier oils. Seal tightly and mix gently.

***Funnel.** A small funnel will make pouring your mixture a lot easier.

***Labels.** When you have created your blend, be sure to label it.

Essential Oils for Beginners

Essential Oils A to Z

This section provides an overview of each type of essential oil along with its characteristics, properties, main uses, suggested blends, and safety precautions.

Essential Oils for Beginners

Allspice

Botanical name: *Pimenta officinalis*

Characteristics: Warm, spicy, and sweet with a strong aroma, similar to cinnamon and clove. It has a thin consistency and as is cocoa-brown in color. Used as a middle note in blends.

Extraction method: Steam distillation

Properties: Analgesic, anesthetic, antibacterial, antifungal, antioxidant, antiseptic, antiviral, aphrodisiac, carminative, rubefacient, stimulant.

How to use: Dilute to desired ratio. May be applied topically or diffused.

Therapeutic uses: Allspice is known to be effective for many types of infections including dental, viral, and bacterial. Also used for digestive issues such as nausea and indigestion. Addition uses include emotional release, calming, anxiety, depression, arthritis pain, muscle pain and stiffness, rheumatism, neuralgia, coughs, and bronchitis.

Suggested blends: Bay, bergamot, black pepper, cistus, coriander, geranium, ginger, lavender, neroli, opopanax, orange, patchouli, ylang ylang

Safety precautions: Best blended in low ratios. At full strength it can be a mucous membrane irritant. May cause skin irritation. Avoid during pregnancy. Contraindicated for those with liver disease.

Note: Christopher Columbus discovered this spice on the island of Jamaica.

Amyris

Botanical name: *Amyris balsamifera*

Characteristics: Gentle, woody mild aroma with sweet vanilla notes. The oil is pale yellow in color and has a thick consistency. It is used as a base note in aromatherapy.

Extraction method: Steam distillation

Properties: Antiseptic, balsamic, decongestant, emollient, muscle relaxant, sedative

How to use: Dilute to desired ratio. Use in diffuser or topically.

Therapeutic uses: Amyris is effective as a decongestant and also for relaxing tight muscles. Additional uses include aphrodisiac, natural fixative, fragrance, relaxation, calming.

Suggested blends: Cedarwood, citronella, ginger, ho wood, lavender, oakmoss, Peru balsam, ylang ylang

Safety precautions: Generally considered safe. May cause skin irritation.

Note: Can be used as substitute for sandalwood.

Angelica

Botanical name: *Angelica archangelica*

Characteristics: Sharp, green, peppery, medium-strong aroma. The oil is pale yellow in color with a thin consistency. Used as a base note in blends.

Extraction method: Steam distillation

Properties: Antibacterial, antifungal, antispasmodic, carminative, depurative, diaphoretic, digestive, diuretic, emmenagogue, expectorant, febrifuge, nervine, stimulant, stomachic, tonic

How to use: Dilute to desired ratio. May be used in a diffuser, applied topically, or ingested.

Therapeutic uses: Has soothing qualities that relax muscles and nerves. Also effective as a digestive tonic, expectorant, stimulant, stress relief, anti-anxiety, fatigue, fragrance, gout, psoriasis, water retention, and reproductive issues.

Suggested blends: Citrus oils, clary sage, oakmoss, opopanax, patchouli, vetiver

Safety precautions: Do not use during pregnancy. Phototoxic properties—avoid sunlight for 12 hours after use.

Note: During the Black Plague, Angelica was used as an antidote.

Anise Seed

Botanical name: *Pimpinella anisum*

Characteristics: Fresh, sweet, spicy licorice-like aroma with medium strength. It is clear and has a thin consistency. Used as a top note in blends.

Extraction method: Steam distillation

Properties: Analgesic, antiseptic, antispasmodic, aperitive, carminative, digestive, diuretic, emmenagogue, expectorant, stimulant, stomachic

How to use: Dilute to desired ratio. May be applied topically, used in a diffuser or inhaled.

Therapeutic uses: This essential oil is effective for fighting colds and flu, bronchitis, coughs, and respiratory infections. Also useful for relaxation and stress relief, muscle aches, and flatulence.

Suggested blends: Bay, black pepper, ginger, lavender, orange, pine, rose

Safety precautions: Do not use while pregnant or breastfeeding. Has been known to cause skin irritation.

Note: Anise seed has been used for centuries both as a spice and for medicinal purposes. It is used to flavor the popular Turkish drink, Raki.

Essential Oils for Beginners

Balsam Fir

Botanical name: *Myroxylon pereirae*

Characteristics: Deep, rich, woody aroma with hints of vanilla, cinnamon, and benzoin. It is dark brown in color and has a thick, almost syrupy consistency. Used as a base note.

Extraction method: Steam distillation

Properties: Anti-inflammatory, antiseptic, astringent, expectorant, sedative, tonic and anticoagulant

How to use: Dilute to desired ratio. May be used in a diffuser or inhaled. Not suggested for topical use due possible skin irritation.

Therapeutic uses: Anxiety, asthma, infections (respiratory, sinus, bronchitis, flu, colds, chronic cough, urinary tract), rheumatism, nervous tension, stress related conditions, wounds, sore and tired muscles, joints and tendons, back pain, sciatica.

Suggested blends: Douglas fir, White fir, spruce, pine

Safety precautions: Can cause skin irritation or sensitivity. Consult doctor if pregnant.

Note: Diffuse during holiday season for a wonderful, Christmas tree scent.

Basil

Botanical name: *Ocimum basilicum*

Characteristics: Sweet, licorice-like, medium aroma. It is clear in color with a thin consistency. Used as a top note in blends.

Extraction method: Steam distillation

Properties: Antibacterial, anti-inflammatory, antiseptic, antispasmodic, carminative, cephalic, digestive, emmenagogue, expectorant, febrifuge, stimulant, stomachic, tonic

How to use: Dilute to desired ratio. May be used in a diffuser, inhaled, or applied topically.

Therapeutic uses: Bronchitis, colds, coughs, dandruff, depression, exhaustion, fever, flatulence, flu, gout, headache, insect bites, insect repellent, insomnia, mental fatigue, muscle aches, rheumatism, sinusitis.

Suggested blends: Bergamot, citronella, citrus oils, clary sage, geranium, hyssop, opopanax, rosemary

Safety precautions: May cause skin irritation. Do not use during pregnancy. Avoid if epileptic.

Note: In Greek, basil means "king of plants." Used frequently in cooking. Considered a sacred plant in India.

Bay Laurel

Botanical name: *Laurus nobilis*

Characteristics: Fresh, spicy, medicinal, herbaceous aroma. Used as a middle note in blends. It is an almost clear oil with a thin consistency.

Extraction method: Steam distillation

Properties: Analgesic, anesthetic, antibacterial, anticonvulsant, antifungal, antimicrobial, antirheumatic, antiseptic, aperitive, carminative, diaphoretic, diuretic, expectorant, sedative

How to use: Dilute to desired ratio with carrier oil of choice. Diffuse or inhale. Use caution when applying topically as it is a know skin irritant.

Therapeutic uses: Amenorrhea, asthma, bacterial infection, bronchitis, colds, flu, rheumatoid arthritis, edema, liver stimulant, gas, bloating, digestive issues, viral infection.

Suggested blends: Bergamot, clary sage, cypress, frankincense, ginger, juniper, lavender, orange, patchouli, pine, rosemary, ylang ylang

Safety precautions: Do not use during pregnancy. Has been known to cause skin irritation.

Note: Also known as laurel leaf.

Bay West Indies

Botanical name: *Pimenta racemosa*

Characteristics: Sweet, spicy, medicinal, balsamic aroma. It is a deep golden yellow in color with a thin to medium consistency. Middle to top note classification.

Extraction method: Steam distillation

Properties: Analgesic, anticonvulsant, antineuralgic, antiseptic, astringent, expectorant, hair tonic, stimulant.

How to use: Dilute to desired ratio. Best for topical use.

Therapeutic uses: Bay is used to treat a variety of skin and scalp conditions including dandruff, hair growth, oily skin, and skin infections. Also effective for rheumatism, neuralgia, muscular aches and pains, circulation problems, colds, flu, dental infections, and diarrhea.

Suggested blends: Bergamot, black pepper, cardamom, cedarwood, cinnamon, clove, coriander, eucalyptus, frankincense, geranium, ginger, lavender, grapefruit, lemon, mandarin, nutmeg, orange, petitgrain, rose, rosemary, sandalwood, thyme, ylang ylang

Safety precautions: Do not ingest internally or use while pregnant. Do not use if you have liver or kidney impairments.

Note: Bay West Indies is often used in men's fragrances.

Benzoin

Botanical name: *Styrax benzoin*

Characteristics: Sweet, warm, vanilla-like aroma. It is golden brown in color with a syrup-like consistency. Used as a base note.

Extraction method: Solvent extraction (ethanol)

Properties: Antiseptic, anti-depressant, astringent, anti-inflammatory, anti-microbial, carminative, cordial, deodorant, diuretic, expectorant, sedative and vulnerary

How to use: Dilute to desired ratio. May be used topically, or in a diffuser or inhaled.

Therapeutic uses: Benzoin is effective against a variety of ailments including arthritis, asthma, bleeding, bronchitis, coughs, colds, wounds, acne, eczema, psoriasis, rheumatism, scar tissue, circulation, nervous tension, stress, muscle pains, chilblains, sore throat, rashes and mouth ulcers.

Suggested blends: bergamot, coriander, frankincense, juniper, lavender, lemon, myrrh, orange, petitgrain, rose, and sandalwood

Safety precautions: Should not be ingested internally. Do not use during pregnancy.

Note: Also known as gum Benjamin. Before synthetically made antiseptics became widespread, benzoin was used for this purpose in hospitals. One of the ingredients traditionally used in incense.

Bergamot

Botanical name: *Citrus bergamia*

Characteristics: Fresh, sweet, floral citrus scent that is both uplifting and relaxing. It is a green to greenish-yellow oil with a watery consistency. Used as a top note.

Extraction method: Cold expression

Properties: Analgesic, anthelmintic, antibacterial, antidepressant, antiseptic, antispasmodic, astringent, carminative, deodorant, digestive, diuretic, expectorant, febrifuge, laxative, rubefacient, sedative, stimulant, stomachic, tonic, vulnerary

How to use: Dilute to desired ratio. May be applied topically or used in a diffuser.

Therapeutic uses: This relaxing scent is great for treating depression, stress, anxiety, tension, fear, and anger. Also used against infections, skin problems, anorexia, psoriasis, eczema, acne, cold sores, urinary tract infections, inflammation, and addictions.

Suggested blends: Black pepper, chamomile, citrus oils, coriander, cypress, frankincense, geranium, helichrysum, jasmine, juniper, lavender, lemon balm, mandarin, neroli, nutmeg, rose, sandalwood, vetiver, violet, ylang ylang

Safety precautions: Generally considered safe. Avoid exposure to direct sunlight or ultraviolet light for 48 hours as bergamot can cause photosensitivity. Consult with physician if pregnant or nursing.

Note: Used as the flavoring for Earl Grey tea. Widely used in the perfume industry.

Black Pepper

Botanical name: *Piper nigrum*

Characteristics: Pungent, dry, and crisp aroma that is both energizing and comforting. Color can range from light amber to a yellowish green and it has a watery consistency. Used as a middle note in blends.

Extraction method: Steam distillation

Properties: Analgesic, antibacterial, antifungal, antimicrobial, antiseptic, antispasmodic, aperitive, aphrodisiac, bitter, carminative, diaphoretic, digestive, diuretic, febrifuge, laxative, rubefacient, stimulant, stomachic, tonic, vasodilator

How to use: Dilute to desired ratio. Can be used topically or diffused.

Therapeutic uses: Helps to relieve digestive upsets including heartburn, diarrhea, and nausea. It is also used to improve circulation and increase muscle tone. Additional used include appetite stimulant, fungal infections, pain relief, rheumatism, chills, flu, colds, dysentery, exhaustion, muscular aches, nerves, and fevers.

Suggested blends: Cardamom, clary sage, clove, frankincense, geranium, lavender, juniper, marjoram, myrrh, orange, nutmeg, rosemary, sage, sandalwood, tea tree, vetiver, ylang ylang

Safety precautions: May cause skin sensitivity. Consult with physician if pregnant.

Note: One of the world's oldest spices. Used in the ancient civilizations of Egypt, Greece, and Rome.

Blue Cyprus

Botanical name: *Callitris intratropica*

Characteristics: Has a light, woody, balsamic scent. The oil is a beautiful blue color with a thick consistency. Used as a middle note. It is soothing and relaxing without having a sedative effect.

Extraction method: Steam distillation

Properties: Anti-inflammatory, antiviral, insect repellent and stimulant

How to use: Dilute to desired ratio. Can be inhaled directly or used in a diffuser. Also used topically.

Therapeutic uses: Used to treat many types of infections including chicken pox, herpes simplex type 2, herpes zoster, yeast infections (Candida), cold sores, flu, mononucleosis, mumps, and other viral infections. May also treat abdominal cramps, muscle aches, athlete's foot, corns, dermatitis, digestion issues, eczema, gangrene, hyperthyroid, immune system, insect repellent, rashes, ringworm, and dry skin.

Suggested blends: Lavender, tea tree, lemon myrtle, geranium, cedarwood, pine, orange, sandalwood, clary sage, juniper, rose, jasmine, and cardamom

Safety precautions: Mild skin and eye irritant

Note: Blue cypress is a natural mosquito repellant.

Blue Tansy

Botanical name: *Tanacetum annuum*

Characteristics: Has a sweet, herbaceous scent. It is a beautiful blue color with a watery consistency. Used as a base note.

Extraction method: Steam distillation

Properties: Anti-inflammatory, analgesic, anesthetic, anti-itching, antihistamine, antibacterial, hypotensive, relaxant, and nervine

How to use: Dilute to desired ratio. May be applied topically, diffused, or inhaled directly.

Therapeutic uses: Allergies, asthma, inflammation, itching, liver cleanser, low blood pressure, lymphatic system, muscle aches and pain, nervous tension, pain, radiation burns, respiratory support, sciatica, skin conditions, sprains, stress and sunburn.

Suggested blends: Lavender, cistus, cedar wood, helichrysum, lavender, ravensara, and rosemary

Safety precautions: Do not ingest, poisonous. Consult with a physician if pregnant.

Note: Also known as Moroccan chamomile.

Cajeput

Botanical name: *Melaleuca minor*

Characteristics: This essential oil has a strong, slightly sweet, camphorous, and medicinal aroma. It is colorless or a very pale yellow with a thin consistency. It is used as a middle note in aromatherapy.

Extraction method: Steam distillation

Properties: Analgesic, antibacterial, antimicrobial, antineuralgic, antiseptic, antispasmodic, carminative, decongestant, diaphoretic, expectorant, febrifuge, insecticide, sudorific, tonic, vulnerary

How to use: Dilute to desired ratio. May be applied topically, used in a diffuser, or inhaled directly.

Therapeutic uses: Helps to calm the digestive system and relieves colic, vomiting, and nausea. Helps skin conditions including acne, rash, psoriasis. Other uses include infections, colds, headache, laryngitis, bronchitis, asthma, sore throat, sinusitis, insect bites, pain relief, tooth aches, gout, and rheumatism.

Suggested blends: Angelica, bergamot, cedarwood, clary sage, cloves, geranium, lavender, marjoram, oakmoss, pine, rosemary, spice oils, thyme, ylang ylang

Safety precautions: May cause skin irritation in some people. Do not use during pregnancy.

Note: Also called white tea tree. Makes a good insect repellant.

Camphor

Botanical name: *Cinnamomum camphora*

Characteristics: The aroma of this essential oil is strong, slightly sharp and camphoraceous with wood undertones. It is a colorless to pale yellow oil with a thin consistency. It is a top note.

Extraction method: Steam distillation

Properties: Analgesic, anti-inflammatory, antiseptic, antispasmodic, antiviral, bactericidal, decongestant, diuretic, expectorant, rubefacient, stimulant, sudorific, vermifuge, vulnerary

How to use: Dilute to desired ratio. This is a strong oil and should be used with care. Can be distilled or inhaled.

Therapeutic uses: Used to treat depression, acne, inflammation, arthritis, aches and pains, rheumatism, bronchitis, coughs, colds, fever, flu, infectious diseases, insect repellant.

Suggested blends: Basil, cajuput, chamomile, citrus oils, eucalyptus, lavender, rosemary, spice oils

Safety precautions: Toxic, poisonous if ingested. May cause skin irritation. Do not use during pregnancy. Avoid if epileptic or have asthma.

Note: Camphor oil is used in Vicks Vapor Rub.

Cardamom

Botanical name: *Elettaria cardamomum*

Characteristics: Cardamom has a warm, balsamic, spicy and strong scent. It is colorless to very pale yellow with a light consistency. Used as a top note.

Extraction method: Steam distillation

Properties: Antibacterial, antiseptic, antispasmodic, aphrodisiac, carminative, cephalic, digestive, diuretic, laxative, nerve tonic, stimulant, stomachic

How to use: Dilute to desired ratio with carrier oil. Can be applied topically, inhaled, or diffused in a diffuser.

Therapeutic uses: Abdominal inflammation, colic, coughs, dyspepsia, flatulence, halitosis, headaches, heartburn, indigestion, lung infection, mental fatigue, nausea, pyrosis, sciatica, sinus infection, and vomiting.

Suggested blends: Bay, bergamot, black pepper, caraway, cedarwood, cinnamon, cloves, coriander, fennel, ginger, grapefruit, jasmine, lemon, lemongrass, litsea cubeba, mandarin, neroli, orange, palmarosa, patchouli, petitgrain, rose, sandalwood, vetiver, ylang ylang

Safety precautions: Generally considered safe.

Note: Cardamom has been used since ancient times. Used by the Egyptians in perfumes and incense. Widely used as a spice in Asian cooking.

Carrot Seed

Botanical name: *Daucus carota*

Characteristics: This essential oil has a dry, earthy, slight sweet aroma. It is pale amber to reddish brown in color with a medium consistency. Used as a middle note.

Extraction method: Steam distillation

Properties: Anthelminthic, antiseptic, carminative, depurative, diuretic, emmenagogue, hepatic, stimulant, tonic

How to use: Dilute to desired ratio. Can be applied topically, diffused, directly inhaled.

Therapeutic uses: Carrot seed is known for helping skin conditions including eczema, psoriasis, dermatitis, oily skin, wrinkles, sunburn, rashes, scars, wounds, burns, and dry skin. Other uses include anemia, arthritis, gout, edema, colic, constipation, diarrhea, eye problems, gallbladder infection, liver conditions, rheumatism, toxic liver, water retention.

Suggested blends: Cassia, cedarwood, cinnamon, citrus oils, geranium, spice oils

Safety precautions: Generally considered safe.

Note: Also known as Queen Anne's lace

Catnip

Botanical name: *Nepeta cataria*

Characteristics: Catnip essential oil has a rich, herbaceous aroma that is mildly floral. It is pale yellow in color with a medium consistency. Used as middle note.

Extraction method: Steam distillation

Properties: Anesthetic, anti-inflammatory, antirheumatic, antispasmodic, astringent, carminative, diaphoretic, insecticide, nervine, sedative, tonic

How to use: Dilute to desired ratio. Can be applied topically, inhaled, or diffused.

Therapeutic uses: Main use is as an insect repellant. Other uses include muscle relaxant, cramps, spasms, gas, detoxification, nervous system tonic, insomnia, anxiety, and relaxation.

Suggested blends: Eucalyptus, grapefruit, lavender, lemon, marjoram, peppermint, orange, rosemary, spearmint

Safety precautions: Do not use during pregnancy. May cause skin irritation.

Note: Catnip has been found to be a more effective insect repellant that DEET.

Cedarwood

Botanical name: *Juniperus virginiana*

Characteristics: This essential oil has a soft, woody, balsamic scent. It is pale yellow to light orange in color and has a viscous consistency. Used as a base note in aromatherapy.

Extraction method: Steam distillation

Properties: Antifungal, antiseptic, antispasmodic, astringent, circulatory stimulant, diuretic, emmenagogue, expectorant, insecticide, sedative

How to use: Dilute to desired ratio. Apply topically, directly inhale, or diffuse.

Therapeutic uses: Cedarwood is beneficial for many skin conditions including acne, oily skin, eczema, and itching. Also helpful for hair loss and dandruff. Other used include anxiety and nervous tension relief, urinary infections, arthritis, and rheumatism.

Suggested blends: Benzoin, cypress, juniper, patchouli, rose, sandalwood, spruce, vetiver

Safety precautions: May cause skin irritation. Avoid during pregnancy.

Note: This oil was used by the Egyptians as part of the mummification process.

Celery Seed

Botanical name: *Apium graveolens*

Characteristics: This oil has a warm, sweet, and earthy scent. It is a yellowish brown liquid with a thin consistency. Used as a middle note in aromatherapy.

Extraction method: Steam distillation

Properties: Antirheumatic, antiseptic, antispasmodic, carminative, digestive, diuretic, emmenagogue, galactagogue, hepatic, nervine, sedative, stomachic, tonic

How to use: Dilute to desired ratio. May be applied topically, inhaled directly, diffused.

Therapeutic uses: Celery is often used for digestive system issues. Other uses include arthritis, rheumatism, gout, joint pain, blood pressure reduction, cholesterol, bladder disorders, kidney problems, cystitis, urinary tract infections, asthma, and cardiovascular health.

Suggested blends: Black pepper, coriander, ginger, lavender, lovage, oakmoss, opopanax, pine, tea tree

Safety precautions: Do not use during pregnancy.

Note: Celery seed is high in vitamin C and calcium.

Chamomile, German

Botanical name: *Matricaria recutita*

Characteristics: German chamomile has a strong, warm, and herbaceous aroma. It is an intense distinctive blue colored oil with a medium viscosity. It is a middle note.

Extraction method: Steam distillation

Properties: Analgesic, anti-inflammatory, antiphlogistic, antispasmodic, bactericidal, carminative, cicatrizant, digestive, emmenagogue, febrifuge, fungicidal, hepatic, nerve sedative, stomachic, sudorific, vermifuge, vulnerary

How to use: Dilute to desired ratio. Maybe used topically, inhaled directly, or diffused.

Therapeutic uses: German chamomile is well-known for its calming and relaxation properties. Uses include anxiety, insomnia, nervous tension. It is also beneficial for a variety of skin conditions: dry skin, eczema, psoriasis, rashes, allergies. Additional uses: menstrual problems, menopause, urinary stones, liver tonic.

Suggested blends: Benzoin, bergamot, citrus oils, clary sage, frankincense, geranium, jasmine, lavender, marjoram, neroli, patchouli, rose, rosemary, tea tree, ylang ylang

Safety precautions: Generally considered safe and non-toxic.

Note: Also known as blue chamomile oil.

Chamomile, Roman

Botanical name: *Arthemis nobilis*

Characteristics: Roman chamomile has a fresh and fruity, apple-like aroma. It is a pale gray-blue in color with a thin consistency. Used as a middle note in aromatherapy.

Extraction method: Steam distillation

Properties: Analgesic, antibacterial, anti-inflammatory, antimicrobial, antineuralgic, antiphlogistic, antiseptic, antispasmodic, carminative, cholagogue, digestive, emmenagogue, febrifuge, hepatic, nervine, sedative, stomachic, sudorific, tonic, vermifuge, vulnerary

How to use: Dilute to desired ratio. Can be applied topically, inhaled directly, or diffused. May also be used as a mouthwash.

Therapeutic uses: Used in children to treat teething pain and colic. Relieves gastric pain, cramping, PMS, diarrhea, abdominal pain. Additional uses: sore throat, allergies, hay fever, asthma, skin conditions, acne, eczema, rashes, dermatitis, itching, dry skin.

Suggested blends: Bergamot, clary sage, eucalyptus, geranium, grapefruit, jasmine, lavender, lemon, neroli, oakmoss, palmarosa, rose, tea tree

Safety precautions: Generally considered safe.

Note: Roman chamomile is often used in soaps and body care products.

Cilantro

Botanical name: *Coriandrum sativum*

Characteristics: Cilantro has a sharp herbaceous scent with faint spicy undertone. The oil is colorless to pale yellow with a thin consistency. It is used as a middle note.

Extraction method: Steam distillation

Properties: Analgesic, anti-inflammatory, antioxidant, antispasmodic, aperitif, bactericidal, digestive, carminative, fungicidal, revitalizing, stimulant, stomachic

How to use: Dilute to desired ratio. May be applied topically, inhaled, or diffused.

Therapeutic uses: Use as a digestive aid. Additional uses: Detoxification, arthritis, colds, colic, diarrhea, exhaustion, flatulence, flu, infections, migraine, muscular aches and pains, nausea, neuralgia, poor circulation, rheumatism, and stiffness.

Suggested blends: Bergamot, cinnamon, citronella, clary sage, cypress, frankincense, ginger, jasmine, neroli, petitgrain, pine, sandalwood, spice oils

Safety precautions: Generally considered safe.

Note: Traditionally used as a culinary herb.

Cinnamon (leaf)

Botanical name: *Cinnamomum zeylanicum*

Characteristics: Warm, spicy distinctive smell. The oil is yellow in color with a medium consistency. Its note classification is base to middle.

Extraction method: Steam distillation

Properties: Analgesic, antibacterial, antifungal, anti-inflammatory, antimicrobial, antiseptic, antispasmodic, aphrodisiac, astringent, carminative, digestive, expectorant, stimulant, stomachic, vermifuge

How to use: Dilute to desired ratio with carrier oil. May be inhaled or diffused.

Therapeutic uses: Can be used for all types of infections such as flu, coughs, and colds; can also help to stabilize blood sugar levels. Other used include digestive problems, viruses, cardiovascular disease, diabetes, ulcers, inflammation, circulation, rheumatism, muscular pain, and warts.

Suggested blends: Benzoin, bergamot, cardamom, clove, eucalyptus, frankincense, ginger, grapefruit, lemon, mandarin, marjoram, nutmeg, orange, peppermint, Peru balsam, petitgrain, rose, vanilla, ylang ylang.

Safety precautions: Do not use while pregnant. Avoid in liver and kidney disease. Do not ingest or apply topically.

Note: Cinnamon oil is a powerful antibacterial.

Cistus

Botanical name: *Cistus ladaniferus, Cistus ladanifer*

Characteristics: Cistus essential oil has a pleasing fruity scent. It is a dark amber in color with a medium to thick consistency. Used as a base note.

Extraction method: Steam distillation

Properties: Antimicrobial, antiseptic, astringent, emmenagogue, expectorant, tonic

How to use: Dilute to desired ratio. Apply topically, inhale directly, or diffuse.

Therapeutic uses: Arthritis, bleeding, boils, bronchitis, circulation, colds, coughs, eczema/dermatitis, fibroids, hemorrhages, hemorrhoids, menstrual conditions, influenza, nervous tension, scars, wounds and wrinkles.

Suggested blends: Bergamot, chamomile, clary sage, cypress, frankincense, lavender, juniper, oakmoss, opopanax, patchouli, pine, sandalwood, vetiver

Safety precautions: Do not use during pregnancy.

Note: Cistus is often used in perfumes.

Citronella

Botanical name: *Cymbopogon winterianu*

Characteristics: Citronella has a fresh, sweet, lemony scent. It is clear in color with a thin consistency. Used a top note.

Extraction method: Steam distillation

Properties: Analgesic, antibacterial, antifungal, antiseptic, antispasmodic, astringent, deodorant, diaphoretic, diuretic, emmenagogue, febrifuge, fungicidal, insecticide, stimulant, stomachic, tonic

How to use: Dilute to desired ratio. May be applied topically, inhaled directly, or diffused.

Therapeutic uses: Most widely used as an insect repellant. Other uses include oily skin, intestinal parasites, and fever.

Suggested blends: Bergamot, cedarwood, citrus oils, geranium, lavender, pine, sandalwood

Safety precautions: May cause skin irritation. Do not use during pregnancy.

Note: Citronella is used extensively as an insect repellant.

Clary Sage

Botanical name: *Salvia sclarea*

Characteristics: This essential oil has a sweet and nutty aroma. It is almost clear to pale yellow in color with a thin watery consistency. Used as a middle note.

Extraction method: Steam distillation

Properties: Antibacterial, antiphlogistic, antiseptic, antispasmodic, aphrodisiac, astringent, carminative, deodorant, digestive, emmenagogue, euphoric, nervine, sedative, stomachic, vulnerary

How to use: Dilute to desired ratio. Apply topically or diffuse.

Therapeutic uses: Clary sage is used for its calming effects and helps with anxiety, depression, nervous tension, and insomnia. Also effective for female reproductive issues including PMS, menstrual cramps, menopause, hot flashes, night sweats, irritability, and heart palpitations. Other uses: muscle pains, kidney disorders, skin conditions, acne, joint pain, and inflammation.

Suggested blends: Bay, bergamot, black pepper, cardamom, cedarwood, chamomile, coriander, cypress, frankincense, geranium, grapefruit, jasmine, juniper, lavender, lemon balm, lime, mandarin, patchouli, petitgrain, pine, rose, sandalwood, tea tree

Safety precautions: Do not use during pregnancy. Avoid when consuming alcohol.

Note: Clary sage has a long history of use for female issues related to menstruation and menopause.

Clove

Botanical name: *Syzygium aromaticum*

Characteristics: This essential oil has warm, powerful, spicy aroma. It is clear to light yellow in color with a thin to medium consistency. Used as a middle note in aromatherapy.

Extraction method: Steam distillation

Properties: Analgesic, antiaging, antibacterial, anticlotting, antifungal, anti-inflammatory, antimicrobial, antispasmodic, antioxidant, antiseptic, antiviral, carminative, expectorant, insecticide, stimulant

How to use: Dilute to desired ratio. May be applied topically or diffused.

Therapeutic uses: Clove oil is an effective pain reliever particularly for cases of toothache, mouth sores, and arthritis. Also useful for respiratory ailments including asthma and bronchitis. Additional uses: acne, burns, cuts and scrapes, parasites, insect bites and stings, vomiting, diarrhea, bad breath, and rheumatism.

Suggested blends: Allspice, bay, bergamot, chamomile, clary sage, geranium, ginger, grapefruit, jasmine, lavender, lemon, mandarin, palmarosa, rose, sandalwood, vanilla, ylang ylang

Safety precautions: May cause skin and mucus membrane irritation. Do not use undiluted. Avoid during pregnancy and with liver and kidney conditions.

Note: Clove has been used for centuries in Traditional Chinese Medicine.

Combava Petitgrain

Botanical name: *Citrus hystrix*

Characteristics: This essential oil has a very strong aroma with woody and citrus notes. It is pale yellow in color with a thin watery consistency.

Extraction method: Steam distillation

Properties: Antiseptic, bactericidal, deodorant, diuretic, emmenagogue, fungicidal, insecticide

How to use: Dilute to desired ratio with carrier oil. Apply topically or diffuse.

Therapeutic uses: Petitgrain is used for its calming properties and works well for easing stress, anxiety, panic, anger, and relaxation. Other uses include insomnia, muscle spasms, acne, oily skin, skin toner.

Suggested blends: Benzoin, bergamot, cedarwood, clary sage, cypress, Douglas fir, frankincense, geranium, myrrh, rose, sandalwood

Safety precautions: Can cause skin irritation. Do not use during pregnancy. Avoid eye contact.

Note: Petitgrain is harvested from orange trees and is an ingredient in eau-de-cologne.

Copaiba

Botanical name: *Copaifera officinalis*

Characteristics: This oil hs a mild, sweet, and woody aroma. It is yellow to brownish in color with a medium to heavy viscosity. Used as a base note in aromatherapy.

Extraction method: Steam distillation

Properties: Analgesic, antibacterial, anti-inflammatory, antiseptic, disinfectant, diuretic, expectorant, stimulant

How to use: Dilute to desired ratio with carrier oil. May be applied topically, inhaled, or diffused.

Therapeutic uses: Used to treat hemorrhoids, diarrhea, urinary tract infections, constipation, bronchitis, sinusitis, skin conditions, sore throat, ulcers, and insect bites.

Suggested blends: Cedarwood, citrus oils, clary sage, frankincense, jasmine, rose, sandalwood, spice oils, vanilla, ylang ylang

Safety precautions: Do not use during pregnancy. May cause skin irritation.

Note: Indigenous to the Amazon rainforest region.

Coriander

Botanical name: *Coriandrum sativum*

Characteristics: This oil has a sweet, woody, spicy scent. It is colorless to pale yellow with a thin watery consistency. Used as a middle note in aromatherapy.

Extraction method: Steam distillation

Properties: Analgesic, aphrodisiac, antispasmodic, carminative, depurative, deodorant, digestive, carminative, fungicidal, lipolytic, stimulant and stomachic

How to use: Dilute to desired ratio. May be applied topically, inhaled directly, diffused.

Therapeutic uses: This uplifting oil can be used to relieve stress, mental fatigue, tension, anxiety, and nervousness. Also good for headache, cramps, rheumatism, arthritis, muscle spasms, cold and flu, and general detoxification.

Suggested blends: Bergamot, black pepper, cardamom, cinnamon, clary sage, clove, cypress, frankincense, geranium, ginger, grapefruit, jasmine, lemon, neroli, nutmeg, orange, palmarosa, pine, ravensara, sandalwood, vetiver, ylang ylang

Safety precautions: Generally considered safe

Note: Used in ancient times as an aphrodisiac.

Cornmint

Botanical name: *Mentha arvensis*

Characteristics: Cornmint has a fresh, minty smell that is somewhat bittersweet. It is clear to pale yellow In color with a thin consistency. Used as a middle note.

Extraction method: Steam distillation

Properties: Anesthetic, antimicrobial, antiseptic, antispasmodic, carminative, digestive, expectorant, stimulant, stomachic

How to use: Dilute to desired ratio. May be applied topically, inhaled directly, or diffused.

Therapeutic uses: Effective for gastrointestinal disorders, flatulence, gallbladder, indigestion, nausea, sore throat, diarrhea, swollen gums, mouth ulcers, and headaches.

Suggested blends: Basil, benzoin, black pepper, cypress, eucalyptus, geranium, grapefruit, juniper, lavender, lemon, marjoram, naiouli, pine, ravensara, rosemary, tea tree

Safety precautions: May cause skin irritation. Avoid contact with eyes. Avoid while pregnant. Do not take internally.

Note: Cornmint is often used in mouthwashes and toothpastes for its fresh menthol scent.

Cypress

Botanical name: *Cupressus sempervirens*

Characteristics: Cypress essential oil has a fresh evergreen scent with balsamic undertones. It is a colorless to pale yellow oil with watery consistency. It is used as a middle note in aromatherapy.

Extraction method: Steam distillation

Properties: Antibacterial, anti-inflammatory, antiseptic, antispasmodic, astringent, deodorant, diuretic, emmenagogue, expectorant, febrifuge, insecticide, sedative, tonic

How to use: Dilute to desired ratio. May be applied topically or diffused.

Therapeutic uses: This is a calming oil which can be used for stress relief and relaxation. Other beneficial used include varicose veins, hemorrhoids, bleeding, nosebleeds, asthma, whooping cough, bronchitis, emphysema, influenza, and menstrual issues.

Suggested blends: Benzoin, black pepper, cedarwood, chamomile, citrus oils, clary sage, ginger, lavender, pine, ylang ylang.

Safety precautions: Do not use during pregnancy. May cause skin irritation.

Note: According to legend, the cross of Jesus was made out of cypress wood.

Davana

Botanical name: *Artemisia pallen*

Characteristics: This essential oil has a rich, fruity, sweet scent. It is a dark green oil with a thick consistency. Used as a base note in aromatherapy,

Extraction method: Steam distillation

Properties: Antiseptic, antiviral, aphrodisiac, disinfectant, emmenagogue, expectorant, nervine, sedative, vulnerary

How to use: Dilute to desired ratio with carrier oil. May be applied topically, inhaled, or diffused.

Therapeutic uses: Davana oil can help to regulate blood sugar levels and used for diabetes. Also used for digestive issues, parasites, infection, anger release, skin infections, headaches, and stress relief.

Suggested blends: Amyris, bergamot, black pepper, cardamom, chamomile, jasmine, mandarin, neroli, orange, patchouli, rose, sandalwood, spikenard, tangerine, tuberose, vanilla, ylang ylang

Safety precautions: Do not use during pregnancy.

Note: Davana oil is said to have a different aroma based on the individual who is smelling it.

Dill Seed

Botanical name: *Anethum graveolens*

Characteristics: Dill has a green, fresh, and grassy scent. It is light yellow and has a watery consistency. Used as a middle note in aromatherapy.

Extraction method: Steam distillation

Properties: Antispasmodic, bactericidal, carminative, digestive, emmenagogue, hypotensive, stimulant, stomachic

How to use: Dilute to desired ratio. May be applied topically or diffused.

Therapeutic uses: Dill oil is often used for digestive disorders including gas, constipation, and hiccups. It is considered calming and can be used to relieve headaches, stress, and nervous tension. Also promotes wound healing.

Suggested blends: Black pepper, caraway, cinnamon, citrus oils, clove, elemi, nutmeg, peppermint, spearmint

Safety precautions: Generally considered safe.

Note: Most famous for its use in making pickles.

Dorado Azul

Botanical name: *Hyptis suaveolens*

Characteristics: This essential oil has herbaceous scent. It is red in color with a medium consistency.

Extraction method: Steam distillation

Properties: Analgesic, anti-inflammatory, antifungal, antimicrobial, antioxidant, anticancer, insecticidal, anti-infectious

How to use: Dilute to desired ratio. Apply topically, inhale directly, or diffuse.

Therapeutic uses: Colds, coughs, flu, bronchitis, asthma, allergic reactions that cause constriction and compromised breathing, any compromise to the respiratory tract, hormone balancer, circulatory stimulant, arthritic and rheumatoid-type pain, reducing candida and other intestinal tract problems, digestion, mouth hygiene, enhances mood.

Suggested blends: Balsam fir, copaiba, elemi, eucalyptus, helichrysum, lavender, wintergreen

Safety precautions: May cause skin irritation.

Note: This is a new essential oil from Ecuador.

Douglas Fir

Botanical name: *Pseudotsuga menziesii*

Characteristics: This essential oil has a crisp, fresh, lemon, evergreen scent. It is clear in color. Used as a middle note in aromatherapy.

Extraction method: Steam distillation

Properties: Antiseptic, antifungal, antitussive, calmative, disinfectant, expectorant, nervine, pectoral, stomachic, tonic, vasodilator

How to use: Dilute to desired ratio. Apply topically, inhale directly, or diffuse.

Therapeutic uses: Used for respiratory infections, asthma, bronchitis, coughs, muscle aches, rheumatism, colds, flu, stress, and anxiety.

Suggested blends: Cistus, fir oils, lavender, lemon, marjoram, pine, rosemary

Safety precautions: Do not take internally. May cause skin irritation. Avoid during pregnancy.

Note: Often used a room freshener.

Elemi

Botanical name: *Canarium luzonicum*

Characteristics: Fresh lemony, balsamic scent. Clear to light yellow in color. Used as a base note in aromatherapy.

Extraction method: Steam distillation

Properties: Analgesic, antiseptic, antiviral, expectorant, fungicidal, regulatory, stimulant, tonic

How to use: Dilute to desired ratio. May be applied topically, inhaled, or diffused.

Therapeutic uses: Used for respiratory conditions including congestion, bronchitis, infections, sinusitis, and coughs. Also used for skin conditions, fungal infections, cuts, and wound healing. Promotes calmness and relaxation.

Suggested blends: Cinnamon, frankincense, lavender, myrrh, rosemary, sage, spice oils

Safety precautions: Generally considered safe.

Note: Often used as a substitute for frankincense and myrrh.

Eucalyptus

Botanical name: *Eucalyptus globulus*

Characteristics: This essential oil has a fresh, sharp, distinctive scent. It is pale yellow in color with a watery consistency. Used as a top note in aromatherapy.

Extraction method: Steam distillation

Properties: Analgesic, antibacterial, antifungal, antineuralgic, antirheumatic, antiseptic, antispasmodic, antiviral, decongestant, deodorant, depurative, diuretic, expectorant, febrifuge, stimulant, vermifuge, vulnerary

How to use: Dilute to desired ratio. Can be applied topically, diffused, or inhaled directly.

Therapeutic uses: Eucalyptus oil is a calming oil that helps boost the immune system. Some helpful uses are for headaches, fevers, respiratory ailments, aches and pains, and skin care.

Suggested blends: Benzoi, cedarwood, chamomile, cypress, geranium, ginger, grapefruit, juniper, lavender, lemon, marjoram, peppermint, pine, rosemary, thyme

Safety precautions: Avoid during pregnancy. May cause skin irritation.

Note: Also known as blue gum.

Fennel

Botanical name: *Foeniculum vulgare*

Characteristics: Fennel has an herbaceous, pepper-like scent similar to anise. It is clear to pale yellow in color with a thin consistency. Used as a top note in aromatherapy.

Extraction method: Steam distillation

Properties: Analgesic, aperitif, antiseptic, antispasmodic, carminative, depurative, diuretic, emmenagogue, expectorant, galactagogue, laxative, stimulant, stomachic, splenic, tonic, and vermifuge

How to use: Dilute to desired ratio. Apply topically, inhale directly, or diffuse.

Therapeutic uses: Commonly used for digestive problems including colic, gas, nausea, constipation, flatulence, hiccups, and vomiting. Additional uses include as a skin toner, for oily skin, and wrinkle reduction.

Suggested blends: Bergamot, black pepper, cardamom, cypress, dill, fir, geranium, ginger, grapefruit, juniper, lavender, lemon, mandarin, marjoram, niaouli, orange, pine, ravensara, rose, rosemary, sandalwood, tangerine, ylang ylang

Safety precautions: May cause photosensitivity. Do not use while pregnant or breastfeeding.

Note: Believed to ward off evil spirits in ancient times.

Fir Needle

Botanical name: *Abies balsamea*

Characteristics: Has a fresh, green, balsamic scent. It is clear in color with a thin consistency. Used as a middle note.

Extraction method: Steam distillation

Properties: Analgesic, antiseptic, antitussive, astringent, deodorant, expectorant, rubefacient, stimulant, tonic

How to use: Dilute to desired ratio. Apply topically, inhale directly, or diffuse.

Therapeutic uses: Used for burns, wounds, bronchitis, coughs, sore throat, sinusitis, catarrh, shortness of breath, arthritis, hemorrhoids, colds, fever, chills, flu, intestinal parasites

Suggested blends: Benzoin, cistus, lavender, lemon, marjoram, orange, pine, rosemary

Safety precautions: May cause skin irritation.

Note: Fir needle was used by Native Americans for several purposes including to speed childbirth.

Frankincense

Botanical name: *Boswellia carterii*

Characteristics: It has a woody, spicy, clean scent. It is clear to light yellow-green in color with a thin consistency. Used as a base note in aromatherapy.

Extraction method: Steam distilled

Properties: Analgesic, antifungal, anti-depressant, anti-inflammatory, antioxidant, antiseptic, astringent, carminative, digestive, diuretic, expectorant, sedative, tonic, vulnerary

How to use: Dilute to desired ratio with carrier oil. Can be applied topically, inhaled, or diffused.

Therapeutic uses: This calming oil is often used to relieve anxiety, promote relaxation, and ease tension. It is also beneficial for respiratory problems including asthma, bronchitis, coughs, colds, and laryngitis. Also used as a skin tonic, for sores and wounds, scar reduction, and rheumatism.

Suggested blends: Bergamot, black pepper, camphor, cinnamon, cypress, geranium, grapefruit, lavender, lemon, mandarin, neroli, orange, palmarosa, patchouli, pine, rose, sandalwood, vetiver, ylang ylang

Safety precautions: Generally considered safe.

Note: Traditionally used as incense.

Galbanum

Botanical name: *Ferula galbaniflua*

Characteristics: Galbanum essential oil has a fresh woody, balsamic scent. The oil is clear in color with a thin consistency. It is used as a top note in aromatherapy.

Extraction method: Steam distilled

Properties: Analgesic, anti-inflammatory, antimicrobial, antiseptic, antispasmodic, balsamic, carminative, digestive, diuretic, emmenagogue, expectorant, hypotensive, restorative, tonic

How to use: Dilute to desired ratio. May be applied topically, inhaled directly, or diffused.

Therapeutic uses: Galbanum makes and excellent skin tonic and is used for acne, boils, cuts, skin inflammation, stretch marks, wrinkles, poor circulation, muscular aches and pains, rheumatism, asthma, bronchitis, catarrh, chronic coughs, digestive cramps, flatulence, indigestion, menopause, PMS and nervous tension.

Suggested blends: Benzoin, fir, geranium, ginger, lavender, oakmoss, pine

Safety precautions: Generally considered safe.

Note: This essential oil is found in many body creams and lotions.

Geranium

Botanical name: *Pelargonium graveolens*

Characteristics: Geranium essential oil has a heavy, sweet, floral scent. It is colorless to pale green with a thin watery consistency. Used as a middle note in aromatherapy.

Extraction method: Steam distillation

Properties: Analgesic, antibacterial, antidepressant, antidiabetic, anti-inflammatory, antiseptic, astringent, cicatrizant, deodorant, diuretic, emmenagogue, hepatic, insecticide, regenerative, rubefacient, sedative, styptic, tonic, vasoconstrictor, vermifuge, vulnerary

How to use: Dilute to desired ratio. Can be applied topically, inhaled directly, or diffused.

Therapeutic uses: This essential oil is a good choice for relieving many skin conditions including eczema, acne, burns, infected wounds, ringworm, lice, shingles, hemorrhoids, and herpes blisters. It also helps to regulate hormones and thus is beneficial for PMS, menstrual issues, and menopause. Additional uses include sore throat, tonsillitis, and edema.

Suggested blends: Bergamot, chamomile, clary sage, clove, cypress, ginger, grapefruit, jasmine, juniper, lemon, mandarin, neroli, palmarosa, patchouli, peppermint, rose, rosemary, sandalwood, ylang ylang

Safety precautions: Do not use during pregnancy.

Note: This is an invigorating oil that can have an uplifting and stress-relieving effect.

Ginger

Botanical name: *Zingiber officinale*

Characteristics: Ginger essential oil has a spicy, warm, and sharp scent. It ranges in color from a pale yellow to dark amber and has a medium consistency. Used as a middle note in aromatherapy.

Extraction method: Steam distillation

Properties: Analgesic, antibacterial, anticoagulant, anti-inflammatory, antioxidant, antiseptic, antispasmodic, aperitive, aphrodisiac, astringent, carminative, cephalic, cholagogue, diaphoretic, digestive, diuretic, expectorant, febrifuge, laxative, stimulant, stomachic, tonic

How to use: Dilute to desired ratio. May be applied topically, diffused, or inhaled.

Therapeutic uses: Ginger is effective for easing nausea, motion sickness, and morning sickness. It is also used in the treatment of arthritis, colds, flu, congestion, coughs, sore throat, diarrhea, cramps, fever, and muscular aches and pains.

Suggested blends: Bergamot, cedarwood, clove, coriander, eucalyptus, frankincense, geranium, grapefruit, jasmine, juniper, lemon, lime, mandarin, neroli, orange, palmarosa, patchouli, rose, sandalwood, vetiver, ylang ylang

Safety precautions: Generally considered safe, however it may cause skin irritation and phototoxicity.

Note: Ginger is thought to have an aphrodisiac effect.

Goldenrod

Botanical name: *Solidago canadensis*

Characteristics: This essential oil has a fresh, spicy, citrusy scent. It is a clear oil with a thin consistency. It is used as a base note.

Extraction method: Steam distillation

Properties: Anti-inflammatory, anti-hypertensive, diuretic, liver stimulant

How to use: Dilute to desired ratio. Can be applied topically, inhaled directly, or diffused.

Therapeutic uses: Goldenrod is often used for liver ailments including hepatitis and fatty liver as well as kidney and urinary conditions. Also used for skin infections, acne, inflammations of the skin, wounds, sores, insect bites, hay fever, allergies, respiratory congestion, sinus infection, nervous stomach, diarrhea, menstrual problems, and impotence.

Suggested blends: Peru balsam, ginger, spruce

Safety precautions: Generally considered safe. Possible skin irritant.

Note: Goldenrod has relaxing and calming effects.

Grapefruit

Botanical name: *Citrus paradisi*

Characteristics: Grapefruit essential oil has a fresh, tangy, citrus scent. It is pale yellow or light pink in color with a watery consistency. Used as a top note in aromatherapy.

Extraction method: Cold pressed

Properties: Antibacterial, antidepressant, antiseptic, astringent, depurative, digestive, diuretic, restorative, stimulant, tonic

How to use: Dilute to desired ratio. May be applied topically, inhaled directly, or diffused.

Therapeutic uses: This essential oil has an uplifting effect making it useful for mood-related disorders such as depression, tension, and stress reduction. It is also an effective skin toner used to treat acne and oily skin. Additional uses include protection against colds and flu, promotion hair growth, athlete's foot, muscle fatigue, cellulite, obesity, liver tonic, increased circulation, and stimulation of lymphatic system.

Suggested blends: Bergamot, black pepper, cardamom, clary sage, clove, cypress, eucalyptus, fennel, frankincense, geranium, ginger, juniper, lavender, lemon, mandarin, neroli, palmarosa, patchouli, peppermint, rosemary, thyme, ylang ylang

Safety precautions: May cause sun sensitivity and skin irritation.

Note: Grapefruit essential oil is an excellent all around detoxifier.

Helichrysum

Botanical name: *Helichrysum italicum*

Characteristics: This essential oil has a strong, earthy, green, floral scent. It is light yellow to red in color with a thin watery consistency. It is used as a base note in aromatherapy.

Extraction method: Steam distillation

Properties: Antibacterial, anti-inflammatory, antimicrobial, antioxidant, antispasmodic, astringent, cholagogue, cicatrizant, diuretic, expectorant, hepatic, nervine, stimulant

How to use: Dilute to desired ratio. May be applied topically, inhaled directly, or diffused.

Therapeutic uses: Helichrysum is well-known for treating injuries to the skin including bruises. It is useful for treating scars and wound healing, dry and cracked skin, stretch marks, warts, and wrinkles. Additional uses include acne, allergies, arthritis, asthma, bronchitis, coughs, muscle aches and p ain, rheumatism, and ulcers.

Suggested blends: Bergamot, black pepper, chamomile, citrus oils, clary sage, clove, cypress, geranium, juniper, lavender, neroli, oakmoss, oregano, palmarosa, rose, rosemary, tea tree, thyme, vetiver, ylang ylang

Safety precautions: Generally considered safe.

Note: Also known as everlasting oil or Immortelle.

Hinoki

Botanical name: *Chamaecyparis obtusa*

Characteristics: It has a pleasing woody spicy scent. The oil is a light reddish-brown in color with a thin consistency. Used as a top note.

Extraction method: Steam distillation

Properties: Antibacterial, anti-infectious, anti-microbial, antifungal, antiviral, antiseptic, astringent, insecticidal, decongestant, mucolytic and relaxant

How to use: Dilute to desired ratio. May be applied topically, inhaled directly, or diffused.

Therapeutic uses: Hinoki essential oil is used for respiratory ailments such as asthma, bronchitis, cough, and congestion. It is also used for relaxation and stress reduction and to ease nervousness and anxiety.

Suggested blends: Cypress, Jasmine, Ylang, Ylang

Safety precautions: Generally considered safe.

Note: Hinoki comes from the Japanese cypress, considered on of the Five Sacred Trees of Kiso.

Hops

Botanical name: *Humulus lupulus*

Characteristics: Hops has a rich, dry, floral aroma. It has a yellow to amber color and thin consistency. Used as a middle note in aromatherapy.

Extraction method: Steam distillation

Properties: Antimicrobial, antiseptic, antispasmodic, astringent, bactericidal, carminative, diuretic, nervine, sedative

How to use: Dilute to desired ratio. May be applied topically.

Therapeutic uses: Hops essential oil is most widely used for its sedative effects. As such it can help with anxiety, insomnia, nervous tension, and stress relief. Additional uses include cramps, migraines, dermatitis, rashes, ulcers, asthma, cough, indigestion, menstrual cramps, and pain relief.

Suggested blends: Citrus oils, copaiba balsam, nutmeg, passion flower, pine, spice oils, valerian

Safety precautions: Generally considered safe. May cause skin irritation.

Note: Hops are well known for their role in beer brewing.

Ho Wood

Botanical name: *Cinnamomum camphora*

Characteristics: This essential oil has a bright, warm, slightly woody scent. It is yellow to amber in color. Used as a middle note in aromatherapy.

Extraction method: Steam distillation

Properties: Analgesic, antiseptic, sedative

How to use: Dilute to desired ratio with carrier oil. Apply topically, inhale directly, or diffuse.

Therapeutic uses: This soothing and relaxing oil is beneficial for anxiety, depression, nervousness, and stress relief. It is also thought to be an aphrodisiac.

Suggested blends: Basil, cajeput, chamomile, lavender, sandalwood, ylang ylang

Safety precautions: Generally considered safe.

Note: Ho wood is similar to rosewood.

Hyssop

Botanical name: *Hyssopus officinalis*

Characteristics: Has a sweet, rich, warm scent. Its color ranges from clear to pale yellow. Used as a middle note in aromatherapy.

Extraction method: Steam distillation

Properties: Antibacterial, antiseptic, antispasmodic, antiviral, astringent, carminative, cephalic, cicatrizant, digestive, diuretic, emmenagogue, expectorant, febrifuge, hypertensive, nervine, sedative, tonic, vermifuge, vulnerary

How to use: Dilute to desired ratio with carrier oil. Can be applied topically, directly inhaled, or diffused.

Therapeutic uses: Can be used to relieve anxiety and fatigue. Also used for viral infections, respiratory ailments, coughs and colds, sore throats, influenza, bronchitis, asthma, colic, flatulence, water retention, and indigestion.

Suggested blends: Angelica, bay, clary sage, geranium, grapefruit, lavender, lemon, mandarin, myrtle, orange, rosemary, sage, tangerine

Safety precautions: Do not use during pregnancy or in cases of epilepsy Do not ingest.

Note: Used in ancient times to protect against the plague.

Idaho Blue Spruce

Botanical name: *Picea pungens*

Characteristics: This essential oil has a woodsy, evergreen, balsamic scent. It is clear in color with a thin consistency. Used as a middle note.

Extraction method: Steam distillation

Properties: Antibacterial, anti-infectious, anti-cancer, anti-inflammatory, antispasmodic, antiviral, antiseptic, disinfectant, expectorant and immune stimulant

How to use: Dilute to desired ratio. May be applied topically, directly inhaled, or diffused.

Therapeutic uses: Arthritis and rheumatism, infections (respiratory and sinus), bacterial infection, bronchitis, cough, decongestant, immune depression, muscle tension, sinus infection and congestion, skin conditions, viral infection and cut and wound healing.

Suggested blends: Balsam fir, bergamot, coriander, frankincense, geranium, myrrh, thyme, ylang ylang

Safety precautions: Generally considered safe. May cause skin irritation if used undiluted.

Note: Blue Spruce needles can be used to make herbal tea.

Jasmine

Botanical name: *Jasminum grandiflorum*

Characteristics: Jasmine has a warm, floral, rich scent. The oil is reddish-brown in color with a medium consistency. Used as a middle note in aromatherapy.

Extraction method: Solvent extraction

Properties: Analgesic, anti-depressant, anti-inflammatory, aphrodisiac, carminative, emmenagogue, expectorant, tonic

How to use: Dilute to desired ratio. Can be applied topically, directly inhaled, or diffused.

Therapeutic uses: Jasmine is a soothing oil that is effective in easing depression and nervous tension. It is also used during labor as it can strengthen uterine contraction. Other used include respiratory ailments such as cough, laryngitis, and hoarseness; sexual dysfunction such as impotence and premature ejaculation; muscle pain, aches, and sprains.

Suggested blends: Bergamot, clary sage, clove, coriander, ginger, grapefruit, lemon, mandarin, neroli, orange, palmarosa, patchouli, petitgrain, rose, sandalwood, ylang ylang

Safety precautions: It is generally considered safe although allergic reactions have noted in rare cases.

Note: Do not use while pregnant. Do not ingest.

Juniper

Botanical name: *Juniperus communis*

Characteristics: Has a fresh, green, fruity scent with a balsamic undertone. It is pale in color with a watery consistency. Used as a middle note in aromatherapy.

Extraction method: Steam distillation

Properties: Analgesic, antimicrobial, antiputrefactive, antiseptic, antispasmodic, astringent, digestive, diuretic, sedative, stomachic

How to use: Dilute to desired ratio with carrier oil. May be applied topically, inhaled directly, or diffused.

Therapeutic uses: Juniper's sedative properties make it an excellent choice for relieving anxiety, stress relief, and calming nervous tension. As a skin tonic it helps clear acne, eczema, oily skin, dandruff, and psoriasis. It is also helpful for digestive issues, fluid retention, bloating, menstrual cramps, gout, arthritis, and rheumatism.

Suggested blends: Black pepper, cedarwood, clary sage, cypress, elemi, fir needle, lavender, oakmoss, rosemary

Safety precautions: Do not use while pregnant or in cases of liver or kidney disease.

Note: Juniper berries are used to flavor gin.

Lavandin

Botanical name: *Lavandula abrialis*

Characteristics: Has a strong, sweet, floral scent. The oil is light yellow with a thin consistency. Used a middle to top note in aromatherapy.

Extraction method: Steam distillation

Properties: antidepressant, antiseptic, analgesic, cicatrisant, expectorant, nervine, and vulnerary

How to use: Dilute to desired ratio. Can be applied topically, inhaled directly, or diffused.

Therapeutic uses: Lavandin oil can be used to relieve anxiety, nervousness, and depression. It also as analgesic properties which make it useful for fighting pain and inflammation in cases such as headache, muscle pain, joint pain, and toothaches. It is also beneficial for the skin, helping to fade acne, stretch marks, boils, wounds, and wrinkles.

Suggested blends: Bergamot, Citronella, Lemongrass, Cinnamon, Rosemary, Pine, Jasmine, Thyme and Patchouli

Safety precautions: Generally considered safe. Avoid during pregnancy.

Note: Lavandin has a powerful scent that tends to overpower others in blends.

Lavender

Botanical name: *Lavandula angustifolia*

Characteristics: Lavender has a sweet floral scent that is highly prized. The oil is clear in color with a thin, watery consistency. Used as a middle note in aromatherapy.

Extraction method: Steam distillation

Properties: Analgesic, antibacterial, anti-inflammatory, antimicrobial, antiseptic, antispasmodic, aromatic, carminative, cholagogue, deodorant, diuretic, emmenagogue, insecticide, nervine, sedative, stimulant, stomachic, vulnerary

How to use: Dilute to desired ratio. Apply topically, inhale directly, or diffuse.

Therapeutic uses: Lavender is a soothing oil which makes it good for anxiety, depression, nervous tension, stress relief as well as headaches, migraine, and insomnia. It is also helpful for respiratory system complaints such as asthma, bronchitis, and colds. As a skin tonic, it is beneficial for acne, boils, burns, sunburn, wounds, psoriasis, bites, and stings. Additional uses include colic, flatulence, nausea, vomiting, arthritis, rheumatism, muscle aches and pains.

Suggested blends: Bergamot, black pepper, cedarwood, chamomile, clary sage, clove, cypress, eucalyptus, geranium, grapefruit, juniper, lemon, lemongrass, mandarin, marjoram, oakmoss, palmarosa, patchouli, peppermint, pine, ravensara, rose, rosemary, tea tree, thyme, vetiver

Safety precautions: Generally considered safe.

Note: Researchers have found that inhaling lavender oil increases beta waves in the brain.

Ledum

Botanical name: *Ledum groenlandicum*

Characteristics: This essential oil has a strong, herbaceous, medicinal scent. It is clear with a thin consistency.

Extraction method: Steam distillation

Properties: Antibacterial, anticancerous, antiviral, anti-inflammatory, antitumoral, nerve stimulant, tonic diuretic and liver protectant

How to use: Dilute to desired ratio. Can be applied topically, inhaled directly, diffused, or taken as a dietary supplement.

Therapeutic uses: Ledum has been used to treat coughs, congestion, fever, laryngitis, colds, and flu. Also effective for liver and kidney detoxification, fatty liver, hepatitis, obesity, skin problems, thyroid regulation, and bloating.

Suggested blends: Celery seed, grapefruit, helichrysum, hyssop, lemon, ravensara, spearmint, wintergreen

Safety precautions: Generally considered safe. Possible skin irritation. Do not use during pregnancy.

Note: Also known as Labrador tea or Marsh tea.

Lemon

Botanical name: *Citrus limon*

Characteristics: Lemon essential oil has a fresh, clean, slightly sour smell. It is pale yellow in color with a watery consistency. Used as a top note in aromatherapy.

Extraction method: Cold pressed

Properties: Antibacterial, antifungal, anti-inflammatory, antimicrobial, antirheumatic, antiseptic, antispasmodic, astringent, carminative, digestive, diuretic, laxative, sedative, vermifuge

How to use: Dilute to desired ratio. May be applied topically, inhaled directly, or diffused.

Therapeutic uses: Lemon oil has a multitude of uses. It is known to boost the immune system and as such helps recovery from colds and flu and other types of infections. It is also good for acne and oily skin, herpes sores, and insect bites. Additional uses include asthma, bronchitis, cellulite, constipation, and headaches.

Suggested blends: Benzoin, chamomile, cistus, elemi, eucalyptus, fennel, frankincense, geranium, juniper, lavender, neroli, oakmoss, rose, sandalwood, ylang ylang

Safety precautions: May cause phototoxicity. Possible skin irritant.

Note: Lemon is a very uplifting oil and can help improve memory and concentration.

Lemon Balm (Melissa)

Botanical name: *Melissa officinalis*

Characteristics: This essential oil has a light, fresh, citrusy scent. It is yellow in color with a thin consistency. Used as a middle note in aromatherapy.

Extraction method: Steam distillation

Properties: Antibacterial, antihistaminic, anti-inflammatory, antiseptic, antispasmodic, antiviral, bactericidal, carminative, diaphoretic, digestive, emmenagogue, febrifuge, nervine, sedative, tonic, uterine, vermifuge

How to use: Dilute to desired ratio. Apply topically, inhale directly, or diffuse.

Therapeutic uses: This refreshing oil can be used to relieve anxiety, depression hypertension, insomnia, and migraines. It is also beneficial for the skin helping with acne, eczema, and as an insect repellant. Other uses include asthma, indigestion, nausea, bronchitis, cough, and cramps.

Suggested blends: Citrus oils, chamomile, frankincense, geranium, lavender, neroli, petitgrain, rose

Safety precautions: May cause skin irritation.

Note: Also known as Sweet Balm and Melissa.

Lemon Myrtle

Botanical name: *Backhousia citriodora*

Characteristics: Strong, fresh, lemon-lime scent. The oil is light to medium yellow with a thin consistency. Used as top note in aromatherapy.

Extraction method: Steam distillation

Properties: Antimicrobial, antiviral, germicide

How to use: Dilute to desired ratio. May be applied topically, inhaled directly, or diffused.

Therapeutic uses: Used to fight infections including colds, flu, fever, viruses, and coughs. Has been shown to be effective against Molluscum contagiosum. Additional uses include acne, oils skin, chest and sinus congestion.

Suggested blends: Bergamot, Eucalyptus, Lavender, Lemon, lemongrass, pine, rosemary, thyme, ylang, ylang

Safety precautions: Avoid during pregnancy. May cause skin sensitivity.

Note: Lemon myrtle is thought to be a more potent germ killer than the more popular tea tree oil.

Lemongrass

Botanical name: *Cymbopogon flexuosus*

Characteristics: Has a heavy, green and lemony scent. The oil is an amber color with a watery consistency. Used as a top note in aromatherapy.

Extraction method: Steam distillation

Properties: Analgesic, antifungal, anti-inflammatory, antimicrobial, antioxidant, antiparasitic, antiseptic, antiviral, astringent, bactericidal, carminative, deodorant, digestive, febrifuge, fungicidal, insecticidal, nervine, sedative, tonic

How to use: Dilute to desired ratio with carrier oil. May be applied topically, inhaled directly, or diffused.

Therapeutic uses: This is a revitalizes oil and as such can be beneficial for fatigue, relieving stress, and clearing headaches. Helpful for respiratory infections including coughs, colds, sore throats, and laryngitis. Other uses include acne, oily skin, athlete's foot, indigestion, and as an insect repellant.

Suggested blends: Basil, bergamot, black pepper, cedarwood, clary sage, coriander, cypress, fennel, geranium, ginger, grapefruit, lavender, lemon, marjoram, orange, palmarosa, patchouli, rosemary, tea tree, thyme, vetiver, ylang ylang

Safety precautions: Possible skin irritant. Avoid during pregnancy.

Note: Lemongrass is highly effective as an air purifier.

Lime

Botanical name: *Citrus aurantifolia*

Characteristics: Lime essential oil has a sweet, citrus, tart aroma. It is pale yellow to pale green in color with a watery consistency. Used as a top note in aromatherapy.

Extraction method: Cold pressed

Properties: Antibacterial, antiseptic, antispasmodic, antiviral, aperitif, astringent, bactericidal, carminative, deodorant, febrifuge, restorative, tonic

How to use: Dilute to desired ratio. May be applied topically, inhaled directly, or diffused.

Therapeutic uses: Lime oil is used as a fever reducer, to boost the immune system and rid the body of colds, flu, and other infections. Also used to treat asthma, bronchitis, coughs, sinusitis, arthritis, circulatory issues, rheumatism, acne, oily skin, and cellulite.

Suggested blends: Citronella, clary sage, lavender, neroli, nutmeg, rosemary, vanilla, ylang ylang

Safety precautions: Avoid sunlight after use due to phototoxicity.

Note: Lime was once used by sailors to prevent scurvy.

Litsea Cubeba

Botanical name: *Litsea cubeba*

Characteristics: The scent of this essential oil is heavy, sweet, and citrusy. It is pale to medium yellow with a thin consistency. Used as a top note in aromatherapy.

Extraction method: Steam distillation

Properties: Antibiotic, anti-infectious, anti-inflammatory, antiseptic, deodorant, digestive, insecticidal, sedative, stimulant, stomachic, vulnerary

How to use: Dilute to desired ratio. May be applied topically, inhaled directly, or diffused.

Therapeutic uses: This oil is an effective remedy in the treatment of acne, oily skin, colds, flu, indigestion, gas, and bloating. Also makes an excellent insect repellant.

Suggested blends: Basil, bay, black pepper, cardamom, cedarwood, chamomile, clary sage, coriander, cypress, eucalyptus, frankincense, geranium, ginger, grapefruit, juniper, marjoram, orange, palmarosa, patchouli, petitgrain, rosemary, sandalwood, tea tree, thyme, vetiver, ylang ylang

Safety precautions: Possible skin irritant.

Note: Also known as May Chang.

Lovage Leaf

Botanical name: *Levisticum officinalis*

Characteristics: This oil has a sweet and spicy yet fresh green smell. It is pale yellow to golden brown with a thin consistency. Used as a top note in aromatherapy.

Extraction method: Steam distillation

Properties: Antimicrobial, antiseptic, antispasmodic, carminative, diaphoretic, digestive, diuretic, emmenagogue, expectorant, febrifuge, stimulant, stomachic

How to use: Dilute to desired ratio. May be applied topically, inhaled directly, or diffused.

Therapeutic uses: Lovage leaf is most well-known for treatment of skin problems such as acne, dermatitis, and eczema, as well as for edema, fever, and menstrual irregularities.

Suggested blends: Bay, galbanum, lavender, myrrh, oakmoss, opopanax, rose, spice oils

Safety precautions: Do not use during pregnancy.

Note: Lovage leaf has been used since the fourteenth century as a medicinal herb.

Mace

Botanical name: *Myristica fragrans*

Characteristics: Mace has a warm and spicy scent. The oil is pale to medium yellow with a thin consistency. Used as a middle note in aromatherapy.

Extraction method: Steam distillation

Properties: Analgesic, antioxidant, antispasmodic, aphrodisiac, carminative, choloagogue, laxative, stimulant, tonic

How to use: Dilute to desired ratio. May be applied topically, inhaled directly, or diffused.

Therapeutic uses: Mace has been used to treat arthritis, colds, constipation, coughs, exhaustion, fever, gas, halitosis, appetite stimulant, muscle fatigue, nausea, and circulatory issues.

Suggested blends: Bay leaf, citrus oils, clary sage, geranium, lavender, lime, oakmoss, rosemary, and neroli

Safety precautions: Do not take internally. Do not use while pregnant.

Note: Mace has been used historically combined with nutmeg.

Mandarin

Botanical name: *Citrus reticulata*

Characteristics: This essential oil has a fruity, light, citrus scent. It is a deep orange in color with a thin, watery consistency. Used as a top note in aromatherapy.

Extraction method: Cold pressed

Properties: Antiseptic, antispasmodic, carminative, digestive, diuretic, hypnotic, laxative, lymphatic stimulant, sedative, tonic

How to use: Dilute to desired ratio. May be applied topically, inhaled directly, or diffused.

Therapeutic uses: The properties of mandarin essential oil make it excellent as skin tonic and beneficial for acne, oily skin, scars, dark spots, and wrinkles. Its sedative properties make it helpful for stress relief, insomnia, and nervous tension.

Suggested blends: Basil, black pepper, chamomile roman, cinnamon, clary sage, clove, frankincense, geranium, grapefruit, jasmine, juniper, lemon, myrrh, neroli, nutmeg, palmarosa, patchouli, petitgrain, rose, sandalwood, ylang ylang

Safety precautions: Generally considered safe.

Note: Traditionally used in Ayurvedic medicine.

Manuka

Botanical name: *Leptospermum scoparium*

Characteristics: This oil has a sweet, rich, herbaceous scent. Used as a middle note in aromatherapy.

Extraction method: Steam distillation

Properties: Analgesic, anesthetic, antibacterial, antifungal, anti-inflammatory, antimicrobial, antiseptic, antiviral, deodorant, expectorant, immune stimulant, nervine, sedative, vulnerary

How to use: Dilute to desired ratio. May be applied topically, inhaled directly, or diffused.

Therapeutic uses: Its most popular uses are for skin and scalp issues. It is known to have exceptional skin healing properties and is good for skin infections of all types including fungal infections, athlete's foot, ringworm, cold sores, dermatitis, itching, and acne. Additional uses include sore throat, muscle and joint pain, dandruff, tonsillitis, anxiety, stress, and insomnia.

Suggested blends: Basil, bergamot, black pepper, chamomile, clary sage, cypress, eucalyptus, geranium, grapefruit, lavender, lemon, litsea cubeba, marjoram, orange, patchouli, peppermint, petitgrain, pine, ravensara, rosemary, sage, sandalwood, tea tree, thyme

Safety precautions: Do not take internally.

Note: Manuka oil is similar to tea tree oil but is milder and potentially more effective against bacterial and fungal infections.

Marjoram

Botanical name: *Marjorana hortensis*

Characteristics: Has a sweet balsamic scent. The oil is clear to pale yellow in color with a thin consistency. Used as a middle not in aromatherapy.

Extraction method: Steam distillation

Properties: Analgesic, antioxidant, antiseptic, antispasmodic, antiviral, carminative, cephalic, diaphoretic, digestive, diuretic, emmenagogue, expectorant, nervine, sedative, tonic, vasodilator, vulnerary

How to use: Dilute to desired ratio with carrier oil. Apply topically, inhale directly, or diffuse.

Therapeutic uses: This oil is helpful for easing tension and calming nerves, clearing congestion, relieving muscle aches and pains, and menstrual disorders.

Suggested blends: Basil, bergamot, black pepper, cedarwood, chamomile, cypress, eucalyptus, eucalyptus lemon, fennel, juniper, lavender, lemon, orange, peppermint, pine, rosemary, tea tree, thyme

Safety precautions: Do not use during pregnancy.

Note: To the ancient Greeks and Romans, marjoram was a symbol of happiness.

Mountain Savory

Botanical name: *Satureja montana*

Characteristics: This essential oil has a sharp, medicinal, herbaceous scent. It is pale to medium yellow in color with a thin consistency. Used as a middle note in aromatherapy.

Extraction method: Steam distillation

Properties: Antibacterial, antifungal, anti-inflammatory, anti-infectious, antiparasitic, antiviral, immune stimulant

How to use: Dilute to desired ratio with carrier oil. May be applied topically or diffused.

Therapeutic uses: This oil has been traditionally used for digestive system problems such as nausea, colic, diarrhea, cramps, and indigestion. It is also effective against viral and and gastrointestinal infections such as colds, flus, shingles, vaginal infections, urinary tract infections, and intestinal parasites.

Suggested blends: Lemon, oregano

Safety precautions: May cause skin and mucus membrane irritation.

Note: Also known as Winter Savory. Has been used as a digestive remedy since the ancient Romans.

Myrrh

Botanical name: *Commiphora myrrha*

Characteristics: This essential oil has a warm, musky smell. It is pale yellow to amber in color with a medium-thick consistency. Used as a base note.

Extraction method: Steam distillation

Properties: Anticatarrhal, antifungal, anti-inflammatory, antimicrobial, antiseptic, antispasmodic, antiviral, astringent, carminative, cicatrisant, emmenagogue, expectorant, fungicidal, sedative, stomachic, tonic, uterine, vulnerary

How to use: Dilute to desired ratio. Apply topically, inhale directly, or diffuse.

Therapeutic uses: Myrrh is helpful for mouth, throat, and gum problems including sore throat, cold sores, gingivitis, and canker sores. It is also effective for skin issues such as boils, eczema, wounds, ringworm, fungal infections, athlete's foot, dry skin, and skin sores. Can be used to relieve menstrual cramps and during childbirth. Additional uses include diarrhea, gas, bloating, and hemorrhoids.

Suggested blends: Bergamot, chamomile, clove, cypress, eucalyptus lemon, frankincense, geranium, grapefruit, jasmine, juniper, lavender, lemon, neroli, palmarosa, patchouli, pine, rose, rosemary, sandalwood, tea tree, vetiver, ylang ylang

Safety precautions: Do not use during pregnancy.

Note: This oil has been used since ancient times for both medical and religious purposes.

Myrtle

Botanical name: *Myrtus communis*

Characteristics: Myrtle essential oil has a fresh, sweet, camphoraceous scent. It is yellow to light brown in color with a thin consistency. Used as both a middle and top note in aromatherapy.

Extraction method: Steam distillation

Properties: Antibacterial, Anticatarrhal, antiseptic, astringent, expectorant, sedative, tonic

How to use: Dilute to desired ratio. May be applied topically, inhaled directly, or diffused.

Therapeutic uses: Myrtle has a long history of use for sore throats and coughs, as well as for chest and upper respiratory congestion. Also helpful for balancing hormones, prostate issues, and skin conditions such as acne, oily skin, and psoriasis.

Suggested blends: Bay, bergamot, black pepper, clary sage, clove, ginger, hyssop, laurel, lavender, lime, rosemary

Safety precautions: Generally considered safe.

Note: Myrtle is considered the sacred plant of the goddess Aphrodite.

Neroli

Botanical name: *Citrus aurantium*

Characteristics: This oil has a sweet, light, floral scent. It is pale yellow in color with a thin consistency. Used as a middle note in aromatherapy.

Extraction method: Steam distillation

Properties: Antibacterial, anti-inflammatory, antiseptic, antispasmodic, aphrodisiac, carminative, fungicidal, sedative, tonic

How to use: Dilute to desired ratio. May be applied topically, inhaled directly, or diffused.

Therapeutic uses: Neroli essential oil's sedative properties make it helpful for nervous conditions such as anxiety, depression, anger, insomnia, panic attacks, and stress relief. Also effective for headaches, heart palpitations, intestinal spasms, colitis, diarrhea, and digestive issues. For the skin, it can reduce the appearance of wrinkles, broken capillaries, and stretch marks.

Suggested blends: Benzoin, chamomile, clary sage, coriander, frankincense, geranium, ginger, grapefruit, jasmine, juniper, lavender, lemon, mandarin, myrrh, orange, palmarosa, petitgrain, rose, sandalwood, ylang ylang

Safety precautions: Generally considered safe.

Note: Also known as orange blossom.

Niaouli

Botanical name: *Melaleuca viridiflora*

Characteristics: This oil has a sweet, camphoraceous, and fresh smell. The color of the oil varies from almost clear to a pale yellow or green with a thin consistency. Used as a middle note.

Extraction method: Steam distillation

Properties: Analgesic, anticatarrhal, antiseptic, antispasmodic, bactericidal, cicatrizant, diaphoretic, expectorant, stimulant, vermifuge

How to use: Dilute to desired ratio. May be applied topically, inhaled directly, or diffused.

Therapeutic uses: This uplifting oil is often used as an antiseptic for wounds, boils, blemishes, cuts, and insect bites. Also beneficial for fighting infections such as colds, flu, fever, bronchitis, pneumonia, whooping cough, sinusitis, sore throat, and laryngitis. Additional uses include intestinal parasites, cystistis, and urinary tract infection.

Suggested blends: Bergamot, eucalyptus, lavender, lemon, orange, tea tree

Safety precautions: Generally considered safe.

Note: This plant is native to Australia and Papa New Guinea.

Nutmeg

Botanical name: *Myristica fragrans*

Characteristics: Nutmeg has a spicy, nutty, and warm aroma. The oil is clear to pale yellow in color with a thin consistency. Used as a middle note in aromatherapy.

Extraction method: Steam distillation

Properties: Analgesic, anti-inflammatory, antioxidant, antiseptic, antispasmodic, apertive, aphrodisiac, carminative, cholagogue, laxative, stimulant, tonic

How to use: Dilute to desired ratio. May be applied topically, inhaled directly, or diffused.

Therapeutic uses: The anti-inflammatory properties of this oil make it helpful for treating muscle aches and pains and rheumatism. It is also a stimulant and good for circulatory problems, digestive stimulant, nauseau, vomiting, and diarrhea. Additionally, it is known to stimulate sexual desire, relieve impotence, and regulate menstrual periods.

Suggested blends: Bay, clary sage, coriander, geranium, lavender, lime, mandarin, oakmoss, orange, Peru balsam, petitgrain, rosemary

Safety precautions: Do not take oil internally. Avoid while pregnant.

Note: Nutmeg is often used in traditional Chinese medicine.

Oak Moss

Botanical name: *Evernia prunastri*

Characteristics: This essential oil has an earthy, dry scent. It is light brown in color with a thin to medium consistency. Used as a base note in aromatherapy.

Extraction method: Solvent extraction

Properties: Antiseptic, demulcent, expectorant, fixative, restorative

How to use: Dilute to desired ratio. May be applied topically or diffused.

Therapeutic uses: Used to soothe inflammation, also good for dry skin, wounds, constipation, and chest congestion.

Suggested blends: Anise, bay, bergamot, clary sage, cypress, eucalyptus, ginger, lavender, lime, orange, palmarosa, tea tree, vetiver, ylang ylang

Safety precautions: Use with caution. Possible skin irritant. Do not use during pregnancy or in cases of epilepsy. Not to be ingested.

Note: This lichen is harvested from oak trees.

Orange, Bitter

Botanical name: *Citrus aurantium*

Characteristics: Has a fresh, citrus scent with a woody undertone. It is yellow to dark orange in color with a thin consistency. Used as a top note in aromatherapy.

Extraction method: Cold pressed

Properties: Anti-inflammatory, antiseptic, antispasmodic, astringent, bactericidal, carminative, deodorant, digestive, fungicidal, stimulant, stomachic

How to use: Dilute to desired ratio with carrier oil. May be applied topically or diffused.

Therapeutic uses: Bitter orange is known for its appetite suppressant properties which in turn aids in fat loss. It also used to stimulate the liver, improve circulation, and treat indigestion.

Suggested blends: Bay, black pepper, citrus oils, clary sage, ginger, lavender, myrrh, neroli, vetiver

Safety precautions: Possible skin irritant. Avoid sunlight due to phototoxicity.

Note: Bitter orange is a key ingredient in many perfumes.

Orange, Sweet

Botanical name: *Citrus sinensis*

Characteristics: Sweet, sugary, citrusy scent. The oil is yellowish-orange in color with a thin, watery viscosity, Used as a top note.

Extraction method: Cold pressed

Properties: Anticoagulant, anti-inflammatory, antiseptic, antispasmodic, bactericidal, carminative, cholagogue, digestive, diuretic, expectorant, fungicidal, stimulant, stomachic, tonic

How to use: Dilute to desired ratio. May be applied topically, inhaled directly, or diffused.

Therapeutic uses: Orange essential oil helps to boost the immune system and is effective for fighting colds and flu and for general detoxification. Also used for constipation, dyspepsia, stress, nervous tension, and insomnia.

Suggested blends: Basil, bergamot, black pepper, cinnamon, clary sage, clove, coriander, eucalyptus, frankincense, geranium, ginger, grapefruit, jasmine, juniper, lavender, lemon, litsea cubeba, marjoram, myrrh, neroli, nutmeg, patchouli, petitgrain, rose, sandalwood, vetiver, ylang ylang

Safety precautions: Generally considered safe.

Note: Oranges are an essential part of Chinese medicine.

Essential Oils for Beginners

Oregano

Botanical name: *Origanum vulgare*

Characteristics: Warm, herbaceous, spicy scent. The oil is pale yellow in color with a thin consistency. Used as a middle note in aromatherapy.

Extraction method: Steam distillation

Properties: Analgesic, anthelminthic, antibacterial, antifungal, antimicrobial, antiseptic, antispasmodic, carminative, cholagogue, diuretic, emmenagogue, expectorant, fungicidal, tonic

How to use: Dilute to desired ratio. May be applied topically, inhaled directly, or diffused.

Therapeutic uses: In studies, oregano has been found to be a very effective pain reliever, and without side effects. For this reason, it is useful for treating arthritis, rheumatism, tonsillitis, sore throat, muscle aches and pains, and headache. Its ant-infective properties make it a good choice for treating respiratory infections, colds and flu, food poisoning, and other digestive infections.

Suggested blends: Bay, bergamot, camphor, cedarwood, chamomile, citronella, cypress, eucalyptus, lavender, lemon, litsea cubeba, oakmoss, orange, petitgrain, pine, rosemary, tea tree, thyme

Safety precautions: Possible skin irritant. Avoid during pregnancy.

Note: Oregano oil may reduce milk supply in lactating women.

Palmarosa

Botanical name: *Cymbopogon martinii*

Characteristics: Palmarosa has a sweet, floral, rose-like scent. This oil is pale yellow with a watery consistency. Used as a middle note in aromatherapy.

Extraction method: Steam distillation

Properties: Antibacterial, antifungal, antiseptic, antiviral, digestive, febrifuge, nervine, stimulant, tonic

How to use: Dilute to desired ratio. May be applied topically, inhaled directly, or diffused.

Therapeutic uses: This makes an excellent skin tonic for fighting acne, dermatitis, dry skin, scars, and wrinkles. It also aids the digestive system and relieves stress, tension, and anxiety.

Suggested blends: Amyris, bay, bergamot, cedarwood, chamomile, clary sage, clove, coriander, frankincense, geranium, ginger, grapefruit, juniper, lemon, lemongrass, mandarin, oakmoss, orange, patchouli, petitgrain, rose, rosemary, sandalwood, ylang ylang

Safety precautions: Generally considered safe.

Note: Palmarosa is native to India and Nepal and has been used there for centuries to fight infections.

Palo Santo

Botanical name: *Bursera graveolens*

Characteristics: This essential oil has a sweet, woody, citrusy aroma. It is clear to pale yellow in color with a thin consistency. Used as a middle note in aromatherapy.

Extraction method: Steam distillation

Properties: Anti-infectious, anti-tumoral, antiviral, antiseptic, anti-inflammatory, immune-stimulant and sedative

How to use: Dilute to desired ratio. May be applied topically, inhaled directly, or diffused.

Therapeutic uses: Palo Santo is known for its use in spiritual practices as well as in meditation and energy work. It can also be used to treat coughs, colds, bronchitis, nasal congestion, allergies, and asthma. Known to be an effective insect repellant and also to get rid of bed bugs.

Suggested blends: Cedarwood, sandalwood

Safety precautions: Avoid during pregnancy. May cause skin irritation.

Note: Also known as Holy Wood. In the same family as frankincense.

Parsley Seed

Botanical name: *Petroselinum sativum*

Characteristics: Warm, wood scent that is somewhat spicy. It is light yellow in color with a thin consistency. Used as a middle note in aromatherapy.

Extraction method: Steam distillation

Properties: Antimicrobial, antiseptic, astringent, carminative, depurative, diuretic, emmenagogue, febrifuge, hypotensive, laxative, stimulant, stomachic, tonic

How to use: Dilute to desired ratio. May be applied topically, inhaled directly, or diffused.

Therapeutic uses: This oil is often used for menstrual regulation and overall uterine health. It can also help with menstrual cramps, nausea, and fatigue. Additional uses include gout, muscle pain, and as a digestive aid.

Suggested blends: Anise, bay, black pepper, clary sage, coriander, ginger, neroli, oakmoss, orange, rose, tea tree, ylang ylang

Safety precautions: Do not take internally or use during pregnancy. May cause skin irritation.

Note: In ancient times, parsley was strongly associated with death.

Patchouli

Botanical name: *Pogostemon cablin*

Characteristics: This essential oil has a musky, smoky, spicy smell. It is yellow to brown in color with a thick consistency. Used as a base note.

Extraction method: Steam distillation

Properties: Antibacterial, antiemetic, anti-inflammatory, antimicrobial, antiphlogistic, antiseptic, antiviral, bactericidal, carminative, decongestant, deodorant, febrifuge, laxative, nervine, stimulant, stomachic, tonic

How to use: Dilute to desired ratio. May be applied topically, inhaled directly, or diffused.

Therapeutic uses: Patchouli oil is one of the best for skin conditions. It helps to quicken wound healing and lessen scarring. It also soothes dry, cracked skin and can lessen the appearance of wrinkles. Additionally, use for acne, eczema, fungal infections, insect bites, sores, and dry scalp. Emotionally, it has a balancing effect and can relieve anxiety, depression, and stress.

Suggested blends: Bergamot, black pepper, cedarwood, chamomile, cinnamon, clary sage, clove, coriander, frankincense, geranium, ginger, grapefruit, jasmine, lavender, lemongrass, litsea cubeba, mandarin, myrrh, neroli, oakmoss, opopanax, orange, rose, sandalwood, vetiver

Safety precautions: Generally considered safe.

Note: Patchouli oil was a popular component of incense during the 1960s.

Pennyroyal

Botanical name: *Mentha pulegium*

Characteristics: This essential oil has a minty, fresh scent. Used as a middle note.

Extraction method: Steam distillation

Properties: Antiseptic, antispasmodic, carminative, diaphoretic, digestive, emmenagogue, insect repellant, stimulant

How to use: Dilute to desired ratio. May be applied topically, inhaled directly, or diffused.

Therapeutic uses: Pennyroyal is often used as a flea treatment for dogs and horses.

Suggested blends: Citronella, eucalyptus, geranium, lavender, lemon, rosemary, sage, tea tree

Safety precautions: Do not use while pregnant. May cause skin irritation. Do not take internally.

Note: Do not use during pregnancy as pennyroyal is a known abortificant. Considered toxic and should be used with great care. Can be fatal in large doses.

Peppermint

Botanical name: *Mentha piperita*

Characteristics: This oil has a fresh, minty scent. Its color is clear to pale yellow and it has a watery consistency. Used as a top note.

Extraction method: Steam distillation

Properties: Analgesic, antibacterial, anti-inflammatory, antifungal, antimicrobial, antiseptic, antispasmodic, astringent, carminative, cholagogue, cordial, digestive, emmenagogue, expectorant, febrifuge, insecticide, nervine, sedative, stimulant, stomachic, vasoconstrictor, vermifuge

How to use: Dilute to desired ratio. May be applied topically, inhaled directly, or diffused.

Therapeutic uses: This uplifting oil helps to fight fatigue, stress, and depression, improves concentration, and clears headaches. It is useful for digestive disorders such as colic, cramps, dyspepsia, gas, and nausea. Use also for the skin-related problems of acne, dermatitis, itching, scabies, ringworm, and sunburn.

Suggested blends: Basil, benzoin, black pepper, cypress, eucalyptus, geranium, grapefruit, juniper, lavender, lemon, marjoram, niaouli, pine, ravensara, rosemary, tea tree

Safety precautions: Do not use during pregnancy. May cause skin irritation.

Note: May reduce milk supply in lactating women.

Peru Balsam

Botanical name: *Myroxylon balsamum*

Characteristics: Sweet, rich, balsamic scent. It is dark brown in color with a thick consistency. Used as a base note in aromatherapy.

Extraction method: Steam distillation

Properties: Anti-inflammatory, antiseptic, cicatrix, expectorant, stimulant

How to use: Dilute to desired ratio. May be applied topically, inhaled directly, or diffused.

Therapeutic uses: Used for respiratory ailments such as asthma, bronchitis, colds, and flu. For the skin, it is used to treat dry skin, cuts, wounds, chapped skin, eczema, and rashes. Also used for parasitic infections.

Suggested blends: Black pepper, ginger, jasmine, lavender, patchouli, petitgrain, rose, sandalwood, ylang ylang

Safety precautions: Generally considered safe.

Note: Peru Balsam is indigenous to Central America.

Petitgrain

Botanical name: *Citrus aurantium*

Characteristics: This oil has a fresh, floral, citrusy scent. It is pale yellow to amber in color with a watery consistency. Used as a middle to top note in aromatherapy.

Extraction method: Cold pressed

Properties: Antiseptic, antispasmodic, carminative, deodorant, nervine, stimulant, stomachic, tonic

How to use: Dilute to desired ratio. May be applied topically, inhaled directly, or diffused.

Therapeutic uses: This relaxing oil will help to soothe anger, anxiety, nervousness, and stress. It also works for insomnia, acne, oily skin, and as a general skin toner.

Suggested blends: Benzoin, bergamot, cedarwood, clary sage, clove, cypress, eucalyptus lemon, frankincense, geranium, jasmine, juniper, lavender, lemon, mandarin, marjoram, neroli, oakmoss, orange, palmarosa, patchouli, rose, rosemary, sandalwood, ylang ylang

Safety precautions: Generally considered safe. Do not use during pregnancy.

Note: This essential oil is used in many perfumes, colognes, and cosmetics.

Pine (Scotch Pine)

Botanical name: *Pinus sylvestris*

Characteristics: This essential oil has a fresh, green, balsamic scent. It is pale yellow in color with a thin, watery consistency. Used as a middle note in aromatherapy.

Extraction method: Steam distillation

Properties: Antimicrobial, antineuralgic, antirheumatic, antiseptic, antiviral, bactericidal, balsamic, cholagogue, deodorant, diuretic, expectorant, hypertensive, insecticidal, restorative, rubefacient, stimulant

How to use: Dilute to desired ratio. May be applied topically, inhaled directly, or diffused.

Therapeutic uses: Use for relief of mental and physical fatigue. Also good for arthritis, gout, rheumatism, muscle aches and pain, asthma, bronchitis, coughs, colds and flu, laryngitis, and sinusitis.

Suggested blends: Cedarwood, eucalyptus, lavender, niaouli, rosemary, and sage

Safety precautions: Possible allergic reaction. May cause skin irritation. Do not use during pregnancy.

Note: Pine was often used by Native Americans.

Ravensara

Botanical name: *Agathophyllum aromatica*

Characteristics: Spicy, woody, camphorous scent. It is clear to pale yellow in color with a thin consistency. Used as a middle note.

Extraction method: Steam distillation

Properties: Analgesic, antibacterial, anti-infectious, antiseptic, antiviral, carminative, diuretic, expectorant, stimulant

How to use: Dilute to desired ratio. May be applied topically, inhaled directly, or diffused.

Therapeutic uses: Ravensara supports the immune system as is helpful for treating infections such as bronchitis, hepatitis, herpes, sinusitis, and shingles.

Suggested blends: Bay, bergamot, black pepper, cardamom, cedarwood, clary sage, cypress, eucalyptus, frankincense, geranium, ginger, grapefruit, lavender, lemon, mandarin, marjoram, palmarosa, pine, rosemary, sandalwood, tea tree, thyme

Safety precautions: May cause skin irritation. Do not use during pregnancy.

Note: This plant is native to Madagascar.

Rose

Botanical name: *Rosa damascena*

Characteristics: Rich, deep, floral scent. It is clear to pale yellow in color with a thin consistency. Used as a middle note in aromatherapy.

Extraction method: Steam distillation

Properties: Analgesic, antibacterial, antifungal, antimicrobial, antiseptic, antiviral, aphrodisiac, astringent, bactericidal, cholagogue, deodorant, disinfectant, diuretic, emmenagogue, hepatic, sedative, stomachic, tonic

How to use: Dilute to desired ratio. May be applied topically, inhaled directly, or diffused.

Therapeutic uses: Soothing oil that is effective for anger, anxiety, depression, fear, nervousness, and stress relief. Helps with circulatory issues, heart problems, and high blood pressure. Useful for female issues such as hormone balancing, irregular periods, infertility, and uterine disorders. Additional uses include asthma, coughs, congestion, nausea, conjunctivitis, eczema, and herpes sores.

Suggested blends: Benzoin, bergamot, chamomile, clary sage, fennel, geranium, ginger, helichrysum, jasmine, lavender, lemon, mandarin, neroli, patchouli, petitgrain, sandalwood, ylang ylang, vetiver

Safety precautions: Generally considered safe.

Note: This is a very expensive oil—perhaps because it takes 40 roses to make one drop of rose essential oil!

Rosemary

Botanical name: *Rosmarinus officinalis*

Characteristics: Fresh, camphourous scent with woody undertones. This is a clear oil with a watery consistency. Used as a middle note.

Extraction method: Steam distillation

Properties: Analgesic, antiarthritic, antibacterial, antioxidant, antirheumatic, antiseptic, antispasmodic, aphrodisiac, astringent, carminative, cholagogue, cordial, decongestant, diaphoretic, digestive, diuretic, emmenagogue, expectorant, fungicidal, hepatic, hypertensive, nervine, restorative, rubefacient, stimulant, stomachic, sudorific, tonic, vermifuge, vulnerary

How to use: Dilute to desired ratio. May be applied topically, inhaled directly, or diffused.

Therapeutic uses: This stimulating oil is effective for boosting memory, clearing mental fatigue, and increasing concentration. It also helps to get rid of headaches and migraine. In addition, it is good for the digestive system including colitis, diarrhea, dyspepsia, gas, and intestinal infections. Other uses include arthritis, gout, rheumatism, muscle pain, varicose veins, bloating, cellulite, asthma, bronchitis, sinus infections, whooping cough, hair growth, and scalp disorders.

Suggested blends: Basil, bergamot, black pepper, cedarwood, cinnamon, citronella, clary sage, elemi, eucalyptus, frankincense, geranium, grapefruit, lavender, lemon, litsea cubeba, mandarin, marjoram, niaouli, oregano, peppermint, petitgrain, pine, ravensara, tea tree, thyme

Safety precautions: Do not use during pregnancy. Avoid in cases of epilepsy or high blood pressure.

Note: Rosemary has been used for centuries. It is referenced by Hildegard of Bingen, the first known herbalist in the Middle Ages.

Sage

Botanical name: *Salvia officinalis*

Characteristics: Fresh, spicy, herbaceous aroma. It is clear in color and has a thin, watery consistency. Used as a top note in aromatherapy.

Extraction method: Steam distillation

Properties: Antibacterial, anti-inflammatory, antimicrobial, antioxidant, antiseptic, antispasmodic, astringent, digestive, diuretic, emmenagogue, febrifuge, insecticidal, laxative, stomachic, tonic

How to use: Dilute to desired ratio. May be applied topically, inhaled directly, or diffused.

Therapeutic uses: Used for menstrual disorders, hormone balancing, infertility, menopause, dermatitis, sores, ulcers, insect bites, and rheumatism.

Suggested blends: Citrus oils, hyssop, lavender, lemon, rosemary, rosewood

Safety precautions: Do not take internally. Avoid in pregnancy or in case of hypertension or epilepsy. May cause skin irritation.

Note: The word sage is derived from the Latin word *salvia*, which means to heal.

Sandalwood

Botanical name: *Santalum spicatum*

Characteristics: This essential oil has a woody, soft, balsamic aroma. It is pale yellow in color with a medium to thick consistency. Used as a base note.

Extraction method: Steam distillation

Properties: Antiphlogistic, antiseptic, antispasmodic, aphrodisiac, astringent, bactericidal, carminative, decongestant, diuretic, emollient, expectorant, fungicidal, insecticidal, sedative, tonic

How to use: Dilute to desired ratio. May be applied topically, inhaled directly, or diffused.

Therapeutic uses: This oil has a calming effect and works to relieve anxiety, depression, fear, insomnia, nervousness, and stress. It is excellent for respiratory problems including infections, asthma, bronchitis, and coughs. For the skin, it can relieve itching, improve dryness, reduce appearance of scars, and for eczema.

Suggested blends: Benzoin, bergamot, black pepper, chamomile, cistus, clary sage, clove, geranium, grapefruit, fennel, frankincense, jasmine, lavender, lemon, mandarin, myrrh, neroli, oakmoss, orange, palmarosa, patchouli, rose, rosewood, tuberose, vetiver, ylang ylang

Safety precautions: Generally considered safe.

Note: Sandalwood is thought to stimulate the production of melatonin, the hormone responsible for sleep regulation.

Spearmint

Botanical name: *Mentha spicata*

Characteristics: This oil has a spicy, minty, and warm scent. It is light yellow to green in color with a thin consistency. Used as a top note.

Extraction method: Steam distillation

Properties: Analgesic, anesthetic, antibacterial, antiinflammatory, antiseptic, antispasmodic, astringent, carminative, cephalic, cholagogue, decongestant, digestive, diuretic, expectorant, febrifuge, hepatic, nervine, stimulant, stomachic, tonic

How to use: Dilute to desired ratio with carrier oil. May be applied topically, inhaled directly, or diffused.

Therapeutic uses: This oil has a stimulating and uplifting effect on the mind making it good for mental fatigue. It is often used for digestive ailments including constipation, diarrhea, hiccups, and nausea. Additional uses include asthma, bronchitis, acne, itching, dermatitis, headaches, migraines, heavy periods, and water retention.

Suggested blends: Basil, benzoin, eucalyptus, jasmine, lavender, lemon, orange, peppermint, rosemary

Safety precautions: This oil is nontoxic and generally considered safe.

Note: This essential oil has been used for centuries and was thought to cure sexually transmitted infections.

Spikenard

Botanical name: *Nardastachus jatamansi*

Characteristics: This oil has sweet, heavy, spicy smell. It is light yellow with a medium consistency. It is used as a base note in aromatherapy.

Extraction method: Steam distillation

Properties: Antibiotic, antifungal, anti-infectious, anti-inflammatory, antiseptic, bactericidal, deodorant, fungicidal, laxative, sedative, tonic

How to use: Dilute to desired ratio with carrier oil. May be applied topically, inhaled directly, or diffused.

Therapeutic uses: This is a calming oil that can be used for anxiety, insomnia, nervousness, and stress. Also good for allergic reactions, migraines, and rashes.

Suggested blends: Cistus, clary sage, clove, cypress, frankincense, geranium, juniper, lavender, lemon, myrrh, neroli, oakmoss, palmarosa, patchouli, pine, rose, vetiver

Safety precautions: Generally considered safe.

Note: Also known as Indian Valerian, Jatamansi, and Nard.

Spruce, Black

Botanical name: *Picea mariana*

Characteristics: Spruce oil has a fresh, woody somewhat sweet scent. It is clear in color with a thin consistency. Used as a middle note in aromatherapy.

Extraction method: Steam distillation

Properties: Antibacterial, anti-infectious, anti-cancer, anti-inflammatory, antispasmodic, antiviral, antiseptic, disinfectant, expectorant, stimulant

How to use: Dilute to desired ratio with carrier oil. May be applied topically, inhaled directly, or diffused.

Therapeutic uses: Black spruce is effective for arthritis, muscle aches and pains, and rheumatism. Additional uses include respiratory ailments, wound healing, and viral infections.

Suggested blends: Amyris, benzoin, cedarwood, clary sage, galbanum, lavender, oakmoss, pine, rosemary

Safety precautions: May cause skin irritation.

Note: Spruce is a refreshing oil that can give a feeling of balance of calmness.

Spruce (Hemlock or Eastern)

Botanical name: *Tsuga canadensis*

Characteristics: Spruce oil has a fresh balsamic scent that is somewhat fruity. It is clear to pale yellow in color with a thin consistency. Used as a middle note in aromatherapy.

Extraction method: Steam distillation

Properties: Antimicrobial, antiseptic, astringent, diaphoretic, diuretic, expectorant, nervine, rubefacient, tonic

How to use Dilute to desired ratio with carrier oil. May be applied topically, inhaled directly, or diffused.

Therapeutic uses: Spruce is helpful for respiratory issues such as asthma, bronchitis, coughs, colds, and congestion. Also effective for kidney and urinary tract infections.

Suggested blends: Amyris, benzoin, cedarwood, clary sage, galbanum, lavender, oakmoss, pine, rosemary

Safety precautions: Generally considered safe.

Note: Spruce was used by Native Americans for spiritual as well as medicinal purposes.

St. John's Wort

Botanical name: *Hypericum perforatum*

Characteristics: This essential oil has a soft, balsamic, herbal scent. The oil clear to pale yellow in color with a thin consistency. It is used as a middle note in aromatherapy.

Extraction method: Steam distillation

Properties: Anti-inflammatory, antimicrobial, antiseptic, astringent, nervine, vulnerary

How to use Dilute to desired ratio with carrier oil. May be applied topically, inhaled directly, or diffused.

Therapeutic uses: This calming essential oil is used for anxiety, nervous tension, and stress relief. It is also effective at relieving muscular aches and pains, headaches, sciatica, arthritis, and rheumatism. For the skin, it is used for minor burns, sunburn, bruises, varicose veins, hemorrhoids, and cuts and scrapes.

Suggested blends: Helichrysum, lavender, wintergreen

Safety precautions: Not for internal use. Do not use while pregnant. May cause skin irritation and photosensitivity.

Note: Unlike the herbal supplement, St. John's wort essential oil is not typically used for depression.

Tagetes

Botanical name: *Tagetes minuta*

Characteristics: This oil has an herbaceous, bitter, green scent. It is yellow to amber in color with a medium to thick consistency. Used as a top note.

Extraction method: Steam distillation

Properties: Antispasmodic, bactericidal, carminative, diaphoretic, emmenagogue, fungicidal, stomachic

How to use: Dilute to desired ratio with carrier oil. May be applied topically, inhaled directly, or diffused.

Therapeutic uses: Effective for bronchitis, congestion, and coughs. Promotes wound healing and makes an effective insect repellant.

Suggested blends: Bergamot, citrus oils, clary sage, jasmine, lavender, lemon

Safety precautions: Possible skin irritant. Phototoxic. Do not using during pregnancy.

Note: Also known as marigold.

Tangerine

Botanical name: *Citrus reticulata*

Characteristics: Sweet, fresh, orange scent. It is a yellow-orange in color with a thin consistency. Used as a top note in aromatherapy.

Extraction method: Cold pressed

Properties: Antimicrobial, antiseptic, antispasmodic, carminative, digestive, diuretic, hypnotic, laxative, stimulant, tonic

How to use: Dilute to desired ratio with carrier oil. May be applied topically, inhaled directly, or diffused.

Therapeutic uses: Good for digestive disorders such as constipation, diarrhea, and gas. Also used for circulatory disorders, fluid retention, and stress relief.

Suggested blends: Basil, black pepper, chamomile, cinnamon, clary sage, clove, frankincense, geranium, grapefruit, jasmine, juniper, lemon, myrrh, neroli, nutmeg, palmarosa, patchouli, petitgrain, rose, sandalwood, ylang ylang

Safety precautions: Possible skin irritant.

Note: Tangerine has many of the same properties as Mandarin essential oil.

Tansy, Idaho

Botanical name: *Tanacetum vulgare*

Characteristics: It has a strong, pungent scent. The oil is a yellow to dark orange in color and of a thin consistency. Used as a middle note.

Extraction method: Steam distillation

Properties: Antibacterial, anticoagulant, antifungal, antiviral, anti-infectious, anti-inflammatory, antispasmodic, analgesic, nervine, insect repellent and stimulant

How to use: Dilute to desired ratio. May be applied topically, inhaled directly, or diffused.

Therapeutic uses: Tansy has had a long use as an insect repellent. In addition, it is effective for a number of skin conditions including acne, dermatitis, eczema, and dryness. Additional uses include arteriosclerosis, hypertension, arthritis and rheumatism, infections, colds and flu, digestive problems, muscle pain, and toothaches.

Suggested blends: Cedar, copaiba, helichrysum, lavender, ravensara, and rosemary

Safety precautions: Do not ingest. Avoid during pregnancy or in cases of epilepsy.

Note: Also known as Cow Bitter, Mugwort, or Golden Buttons.

Tarragon

Botanical name: *Artemisia dracunculus*

Characteristics: Spicy-sweet, green scent. Used as a middle note in aromatherapy.

Extraction method: Steam distillation

Properties: Antiseptic, antispasmodic, aperitif, carminative, digestive, diuretic, emmenagogue, hypnotic, stimulant, stomachic, vermifuge

How to use: Dilute to desired ratio with carrier oil. May be applied topically, inhaled directly, or diffused.

Therapeutic uses: Traditionally used for digestive conditions such as indigestion, hiccups, nausea, parasites, and vomiting. Also effective in treating menstrual problems and urinary tract infections.

Suggested blends: Basil, cistus, galbanum, lavender, oakmoss, pine, vanilla

Safety precautions: Do not use during pregnancy. Do not take internally.

Note: Also known as Dragon's wort and Estragon.

Tea Tree

Botanical name: *Melaleuca alternifolia*

Characteristics: Tea tree has fresh, warm camphoraceous scent. This oil is clear in color with a watery consistency. Used as a middle note.

Extraction method: Steam distillation

Properties: Analgesic, antibacterial, antifungal, anti-inflammatory, antimicrobial, antiparasitic, antiseptic, antiviral, decongestant, deodorant, diaphoretic, expectorant, fungicidal, immune stimulant, insecticide, vulnerary

How to use: Dilute to desired ratio with carrier oil. May be applied topically, inhaled directly, or diffused.

Therapeutic uses: Very effective against all types of infections including colds and flu, cold sores, fungal infections, and fever. Also works on the respiratory system to ease coughs, congestion, asthma, sinus infection, and whooping cough. Additional uses include acne, athlete's foot, burns, rashes, warts, sunburn, wound healing, and dandruff.

Suggested blends: Basil, bergamot, black pepper, chamomile german, clary sage, clove, cypress, eucalyptus, geranium, juniper, lavender, lemon, marjoram, nutmeg, oakmoss, oregano, peppermint, pine, ravensara, rosemary, thyme, ylang ylang

Safety precautions: Do not take internally. Possible skin irritant.

Note: Also known as Melaleuca.

Thyme

Botanical name: *Thymus vulgari*

Characteristics: Strong, spicy, herbaceous scent. It is reddish-brown in color with a medium consistency. Used as a middle note in aromatherapy.

Extraction method: Steam distillation

Properties: Analgesic, anthelminthic, antibacterial, antifungal, anti-inflammatory, antimicrobial, antioxidant, antiseptic, antispasmodic, antiviral, bactericidal, carminative, cell proliferant, deodorant, diuretic, emmenagogue, expectorant, insecticide, parasiticide, rubefacient, stimulant, tonic, vermifuge

How to use: Dilute to desired ratio with carrier oil. May be applied topically or diffused.

Therapeutic uses: Thyme essential oil has a stimulating effect on the nervous system which makes it effective for depression, fatigue, memory boosting, and concentration. Also works on the respiratory system to help with asthma, colds, coughs, laryngitis, sore throat, tonsillitis, and whooping cough. Additional uses include arthritis, gout, muscle aches, rheumatism, sprains, and menstrual problems.

Suggested blends: Bergamot, clary sage, cypress, eucalyptus, geranium, grapefruit, lavender, lemon, lemon balm, marjoram, Peru balsam, pine, rosemary, tea tree

Safety precautions: May cause skin irritation. Do not use during pregnancy or while breastfeeding.

Note: Thyme is one of the oldest medicinally used plants.

Tumeric

Botanical name: *Curcuma longa*

Characteristics: This essential oil has a spicy, woody aroma. It is yellow-orange in color with a thin consistency. Used as a base note in aromatherapy.

Extraction method: Steam distillation

Properties: Analgesic, antiarthritic, anti-inflammatory, antifungal, antioxidant, cholagogue, digestive, diuretic, insecticidal, stimulant

How to use: Dilute to desired ratio with carrier oil. May be applied topically, inhaled directly, or diffused.

Therapeutic uses: Tumeric is effective for digestive disorders including abdominal cramping, indigestion, nausea, and vomiting. It also has anti-inflammatory and pain-relieving qualities which make it useful for conditions such as arthritis, muscle aches and pains, and rheumatism. Studies have shown that tumeric may be useful in cases of Alzheimer's disease.

Suggested blends: Cistus, clary sage, ginger, ylang ylang

Safety precautions: Do not take internally. Possible skin irritant. Do not use during pregnancy.

Note: This spice is well known in Asian cooking and is a key ingredient in curries.

Valerian

Botanical name: *Valeriana officinalis*

Characteristics: Musky, woody, balsamic scent. It is a light brown to reddish brown oil with a medium consistency. Used as a base note.

Extraction method: Solvent extraction

Properties: Antispasmodic, bactericidal, carminative, diuretic, hypnotic, hypotensive, regulator, sedative, stomachic

How to use: Dilute to desired ratio with carrier oil. May be applied topically, inhaled directly, or diffused.

Therapeutic uses: Valerian is a calming oil that is effective for anxiety, depression, insomnia, hyperactivity, nervousness, panic attacks, stress, and tension headaches. Other uses include fever, menstrual cramps, restless leg syndrome, spasms, and tendonitis.

Suggested blends: Cedarwood, lavender, mandarin, oakmoss, patchouli, petitgrain, pine, rosemary

Safety precautions: May cause skin irritation.

Note: Valerian is popular as a natural sedative.

Vanilla

Botanical name: *Vanilla planifolia*

Characteristics: Sweet, rich balsamic scent. It is deep brown in color with a thick consistency. Used as a base note in aromatherapy.

Extraction method: Solvent extraction

Properties: Analgesic, antibacterial, anticonvulsive, antidepressant, antidiuretic, antipyretic, antispasmodic, carminative, diuretic, febrifuge, hepatic, hypotensor, nervine, sedative, stomachic, tonic(nerves), tranquilizer, vermifuge

How to use: Dilute to desired ratio with carrier oil. May be applied topically, inhaled directly, or diffused.

Therapeutic uses: Vanilla is a relaxing oil that can be used to ease anxiety, depression, insomnia, nervousness, and stress. It is also known to be an aphrodisiac and promote sexual arousal. Additional uses include hemorrhoids, infections, menstrual regulation, and varicose veins.

Suggested blends: Benzoin, bergamot, frankincense, jasmine, lemon, mandarin, opopanax, orange, patchouli, rose, sandalwood, vetiver, ylang ylang

Safety precautions: Do not ingest. Avoid during pregnancy.

Note: Vanilla is widely used as in the fragrance and food industries.

Vetiver

Botanical name: *Vetiveria zizanoides*

Characteristics: This essential oil has a heavy, earthy, woody scent. Amber to reddish brown in color with a thick consistency. Used as a base note.

Extraction method: Steam distillation

Properties: Analgesic, antibacterial, antifungal, anti-inflammatory, antimicrobial, antioxidant, antiseptic, antispasmodic, cell proliferant, depurative, emmenagogue, rubefacient, sedative, stimulant, tonic, vermifuge, vulnerary

How to use: Dilute to desired ratio with carrier oil. May be applied topically, inhaled directly, or diffused.

Therapeutic uses: Calming effect which helps with ADHD, anger, anxiety, autism, insomnia, nervousness, and stress relief. Also good for arthritis, muscle aches, and rheumatism.

Suggested blends: Bergamot, black pepper, cedarwood, clary sage, geranium, ginger, grapefruit, jasmine, lavender, lemon, lemongrass, litsea cubeba, mandarin, oakmoss, opopanax, orange, patchouli, rose, sandalwood, ylang ylang

Safety precautions: Generally considered safe.

Note: This essential oil from India has been called the Oil of Tranquility.

Wintergreen

Botanical name: *Gaultheria procumbens*

Characteristics: This oil has a strong, minty, woody scent. It is clear to pale yellow in color with a thin consistency.

Extraction method: Steam distillation

Properties: Antispasmodic, anti-inflammatory, antirheumatic, antiseptic, analgesic, disinfectant, anticoagulant, vasodilator

How to use: Dilute to desired ratio. May be applied topically.

Therapeutic uses: Wintergreen is effective against headache, toothache, muscle aches and pains, arthritis, rheumatism, and other inflammatory conditions. For the skin, it can help with acne, dermatitis, eczema, and wounds.

Suggested blends: Oregano, peppermint, thyme, ylang ylang

Safety precautions: Do not use if pregnant or in cases of pregnancy. Should not be combined with blood thinners such as warfarin. Possible skin irritant. Potentially toxic.

Note: Contains methyl salicylate, the active component in aspirin. Use with extreme caution.

Yarrow

Botanical name: *Achillea millefolium*

Characteristics: Yarrow essential oil has a dry, herbal aroma. It is pale to dark blue in color with a thin consistency. Used as a top note in aromatherapy.

Extraction method: Steam distillation

Properties: Anti-inflammatory, antiarthritic, antibacterial, antifungal, antipyretic, antiseptic, antispasmodic, astringent, carminative, diaphoretic, digestive, emmenagogue, expectorant, febrifuge, stimulant, stomachic, tonic, vulnerary

How to use: Dilute to desired ratio. May be applied topically, inhaled directly, or diffused.

Therapeutic uses: Yarrow essential oil is effective for relieving menstrual irregularities and cramps, constipation, cuts, and wound healing. May also be used for colds, flu, fever, acne, oily skin, varicose veins, and hemorrhoids.

Suggested blends: Angelica root, bay, black pepper, bergamot, cedarwood, chamomile, clary sage, cypress, grapefruit, helichrysum, lavender, neroli, oakmoss, pine, rosemary, valerian, vetiver, ylang ylang

Safety precautions: Do not use during pregnancy.

Note: Yarrow has been used since ancient times for wound healing.

Ylang Ylang

Botanical name: *Cananga odorata*

Characteristics: This essential oil has a sweet, floral, rich aroma. It is a pale yellow in color with a thin consistency. Used as a base note in aromatherapy.

Extraction method: Steam distillation

Properties: Antibacterial, antidepressant, antifungal, anti-inflammatory, antiseptic, antispasmodic, aphrodisiac, cell proliferant, disinfectant, expectorant, nervine, sedative, vulnerary

How to use: Dilute to desired ratio. May be applied topically, inhaled directly, or diffused.

Therapeutic uses: This oil has a soothing, sedative effect on the nervous system making it useful for anxiety, fear, panic attacks, nervousness, and stress. Also used for infections, high blood pressure, dry skin, hair growth, and scalp problems.

Suggested blends: Bergamot, chamomile, clary sage, clove, eucalyptus lemon, ginger, grapefruit, jasmine, lemon, litsea cubeba, mandarin, neroli, opopanax, orange, palmarosa, patchouli, Peru balsam, petitgrain, rose, rosewood, sandalwood, tuberose, vetiver

Safety precautions: Do not use during pregnancy.

Note: The name ylang ylang means "flower of flower."

Recipes

Mood Enhancement

Essential oils are well known for their mood-enhancing properties.

Anger

This mix cools and soothes angry feelings.

Blend:

5 drops lavender

5 drops geranium

5 drops clary sage

1 ounce carrier oil

Directions:

Combine the oils together and pour into a glass bottle with roller top. Roll the bottle slowly back and forth to mix.

Apply mixture to temples, wrists, behind ears, and bottom of feet.

Can also be diffused.

Anxiety

This anti-anxiety blend has a relaxing effect on the nervous system.

Blend:

15 drops lavender

12 drops vetiver

8 drops orange

8 drops frankincense

5 drops copaiba

1 ounce carrier oil

Directions:

Combine the oils together and pour into a glass bottle with roller top. Roll the bottle slowly back and forth to mix.

Apply mixture to temples, wrists, behind ears, and bottom of feet.

Can also be diffused.

Confidence

This is a good blend to try when you need a little boost to your self-confidence.

Blend:

10 drops orange

10 drops of grapefruit

5 drops jasmine

1 ounce carrier oil

Directions:

Combine the oils together and pour into a glass bottle with roller top. Roll the bottle slowly back and forth to mix.

Apply mixture to temples, wrists, behind ears, and bottom of feet.

Can also be diffused.

Depression

This uplifting blend can help fight depression as well as mid-winter blues.

Blend:

5 drops rose

10 drops sandalwood

2 drops lemon

1 ounce carrier oil

Directions:

Combine the oils together and pour into a glass bottle with roller top. Roll the bottle slowly back and forth to mix.

Apply mixture to temples, wrists, behind ears, and bottom of feet.

Can also be diffused.

Energy

When you're felling fatigued and need an energetic pick-me-up, try this blend instead of a cup of coffee.

Blend:

10 drops peppermint

5 drops frankincense

5 drops grapefruit

1 ounce carrier oil

Directions:

Combine the oils together and pour into a glass bottle with roller top. Roll the bottle slowly back and forth to mix.

Apply mixture to temples, wrists, behind ears, and bottom of feet.

Can also be diffused.

Fear

. . . .

Fearful situations can trigger the fight-or-flight response and the release of cortisol. Use this blend to ease this response.

Blend:

8 drops clary sage

8 drops Roman chamomile

4 drops vetiver

1 ounce carrier oil

Directions:

Combine the oils together and pour into a glass bottle with roller top. Roll the bottle slowly back and forth to mix.

Apply mixture to temples, wrists, behind ears, and bottom of feet.

Can also be diffused.

Grief

This blend can help alleviate the painful feeling of grief.

Blend:

5 drops rose

5 drops cypress

5 drops helichrysum

3 drops frankincense

1 ounce carrier oil

Directions:

Combine the oils together and pour into a glass bottle with roller top. Roll the bottle slowly back and forth to mix.

Apply mixture to temples, wrists, behind ears, and bottom of feet.

Can also be diffused.

Happiness

The aroma of citrus oils can increase feelings of happiness.

Blend:

10 drops orange

10 drops grapefruit

5 drops neroli

1 ounce carrier oil

Directions:

Combine the oils together and pour into a glass bottle with roller top. Roll the bottle slowly back and forth to mix.

Apply mixture to temples, wrists, behind ears, and bottom of feet.

Can also be diffused.

Insecurity

Use this blend to boost your self-esteem in times of uncertainty.

Blend:

8 drops cedarwood

8 drops bergamot

4 drops sandalwood

1 ounce carrier oil

Directions:

Combine the oils together and pour into a glass bottle with roller top. Roll the bottle slowly back and forth to mix.

Apply mixture to temples, wrists, behind ears, and bottom of feet.

Can also be diffused.

Irritation

Soothe the feelings of frustration and irritation with this calming blend.

Blend:

10 drops lavender

5 drops neroli

5 drops mandarin

5 drops sandalwood

1 ounce carrier oil

Directions:

Combine the oils together and pour into a glass bottle with roller top. Roll the bottle slowly back and forth to mix.

Apply mixture to temples, wrists, behind ears, and bottom of feet.

Can also be diffused.

Panic

Overcome feelings of panic with this powerful blend.

Blend:

10 drops lavender

5 drops valor

5 drops orange

5 drops Idaho blue spruce

3 drops copaiba

3 drops frankincense

1 ounce carrier oil

Directions:

Combine the oils together and pour into a glass bottle with roller top. Roll the bottle slowly back and forth to mix.

Apply mixture to temples, wrists, behind ears, and bottom of feet.

Can also be diffused.

Stress Relief

The ability to manage stress is very important in today's fast-paced world. The following essential oil blends can help you deal with everyday tension and stress.

Herbal De-Stress

This blend will help you de-stress while also staying alert.

Blend:

10 drops clary sage

5 drops lemon

5 drops lavender

1 ounce carrier oil

Directions:

Combine the oils together and pour into a glass bottle with roller top. Roll the bottle slowly back and forth to mix.

Apply mixture to temples, wrists, behind ears, and bottom of feet.

Can also be diffused.

Serenity Blend

. . . .

The scents of orange and patchouli combine in this calming blend.

Blend:

12 drops ylang ylang

6 drops orange

15 drops patchouli

5 drops bergamot

1 ounce carrier oil

Directions:

Combine the oils together and pour into a glass bottle with roller top. Roll the bottle slowly back and forth to mix.

Apply mixture to temples, wrists, behind ears, and bottom of feet.

Can also be diffused.

De-Stressing Mister

A few sprays of this relaxing blend will help you unwind after a hectic day.

Blend:

20 drops lavender

20 drops clary sage

20 drops rose

4 ounces water

Directions:

Combine all ingredients together in a spray bottle.

Spritz on skin.

Unwinding Bath Oil

The soothing power of warm water combined with this essential oil blend is sure to conquer your stress.

Blend:

10 drops Roman chamomile

10 drops geranium

10 drops frankincense

2 ounces carrier oil

Directions:

Combine the oils together in a glass bottle. Roll between hands to mix. Pour about 1/4 into a bathtub of warm water. Store remaining oil for later use.

Soak for up to 30 minutes.

Headaches

There can be many reasons for headaches, but what they all have in common is that they are painful. Fight a headache with these essential oil blends.

Stress Headache Fighter

A headache is a surefire way to ruin your mood and keep you from doing what needs to be done. Reach for this mix instead of a bottle of Tylenol for quick relief.

Blend:

15 drops peppermint

10 drops eucalyptus

10 drops cajeput

8 drops rosemary

8 drops lavender

5 drops Roman chamomile

1 ounce carrier oil

Directions:

Combine the oils together and pour into a glass bottle with roller top or dropper. Roll the bottle slowly back and forth to mix.

Apply mixture to temples, wrists, behind ears, and bottom of feet.

Can also be diffused.

Migraine Headache Fighter

Put out a migraine fast with this powerful blend.

Blend:

10 drops frankincense

10 drops balsam fir

10 drops copaiba

1 ounce carrier oil

Directions:

Combine the oils together and pour into a glass bottle with roller top or dropper. Roll the bottle slowly back and forth to mix.

Apply mixture to temples, wrists, behind ears, and bottom of feet.

Can also be diffused.

Colds and Flu

Colds and flu can weaken the body and spread germs. Essential oils can be used to fight germs and improve the immune system.

Head Cold Fighter

Oregano is a powerful, natural antiviral.

Blend:

10 drops oregano

10 drops frankincense

5 drops peppermint

1 ounce carrier oil

Directions:

Combine the oils together and pour into a glass bottle with roller top or dropper. Roll the bottle slowly back and forth to mix.

Apply mixture to temples, wrists, behind ears, and bottom of feet.

Can also be diffused or steam inhaled.

Chest Cold Fighter Rub

The powerful scents of camphor and menthol will help to clear out congested nasal passages.

Blend:

15 drops tea tree

10 drops eucalyptus

5 drops peppermint

1 ounce carrier oil

Directions:

Combine the oils together and pour into a glass bottle. Roll the bottle slowly back and forth to mix.

Apply to chest and massage into skin.

Flu and Fever Reducer

Blend:

10 drops lavender

5 drops peppermint

1 cup ice water

Directions:

Combine the oils together and pour into bowl filled with ice water. Swish bowl to mix.

Submerge wash cloth into the solution and then wring out excess. Apply cloth to forehead.

Insomnia and Sleep Disorders

Proper sleep is necessary for good health. Unfortunately many people cannot get the sleep that they need. Place this essential oil mixture in a diffuser or with water as a linen spray for a good night's rest.

A Good Night's Rest

Blend:

5 drops Roman chamomile

3 drops clary sage

3 drops bergamot

1 ounce carrier oil

Directions:

Combine the oils together and pour into a glass bottle. Roll the bottle slowly back and forth to mix.

Apply mixture to temples, wrists, behind ears, and bottom of feet.

Alternatively, add mixture to spray bottle with water and mist pillow before sleep.

Skin and Hair Care

Essential oils are excellent additions to skin and hair care products. Essential oils can keep skin and hair looking and feeling healthy as well as help with specific skin conditions.

Lavender Skin Toner

This toner will leave your skin feeling refreshed.

Blend:

3 drops lavender

1 drops rose

1 drops rosewood

8 ounces distilled water

Directions:

Pour water into glass bottle and add essential oils. Shake gently to mix.

Apply tone to skin with cotton ball.

Cuts and Burns

Help minor cuts and burns heal with an essential oil blend made with healing tea tree oil. Add to coconut oil or cocoa butter for the best results.

Blend:

10 drops lavender

10 drops tea tree

1 ounce carrier oil

Directions:

Combine the oils together and pour into a glass bottle with roller top or dropper. Roll the bottle slowly back and forth to mix.

Apply to wounds twice per day.

Insect Bites, Rashes, etc.

This mixture can help relieve the sting of insect bites and itchy rashes.

Blend:

10 drops lavender

4 drops frankincense

6 drops tea tree

1 ounce carrier oil

Directions:

Combine the oils together and pour into a glass bottle with roller top or dropper. Roll the bottle slowly back and forth to mix.

Apply to bites or rash twice daily.

Athlete's Foot Reliever

This stubborn fungal infection can be difficult to get rid of. Try this tea tree oil blend for faster relief.

Blend:

5 drops tea tree

4 drops eucalyptus

3 drops myrrh

3 drops thyme

1 ounce carrier oil

Directions:

Combine the oils together and pour into a glass bottle. Roll the bottle slowly back and forth to mix.

Apply 1 or 2 drops to affected area twice daily. May take several weeks to clear.

Acne

This acne fighter is tough on acne but gentle on your skin.

Blend:

8 drops lavender

6 drops lemongrass

3 drops geranium

1 ounce carrier oil

Directions:

Combine the oils together and pour into a glass bottle. Roll the bottle slowly back and forth to mix.

Apply a couple of drops directly to affected area in the morning and night after cleansing. Avoid contact with eyes, nose, and mouth.

Skin Brightener

This refreshing lemony blend will tighten pores and lighten dark spots.

Blend:

8 drops lemon

8 drops lavender

4 ounces distilled water

Directions:

Combine the oils together and pour into a glass bottle. Roll the bottle slowly back and forth to mix.

Apply to skin with cotton ball after cleansing.

Minty Sugar Scrub

This invigorating blend will exfoliate your skin and leave your feeling refreshed.

Blend:

4 ounces raw sugar

1 ounce carrier oil

12 drops peppermint

8 drops orange

Directions:

Combine the sugar with the oils in a bowl.

Apply 2-3 tablespoons of mixture to damp skin and massage gently in circular motion. Rinse with cool water. Avoid eyes, nose, and mouth.

Store mixture in glass jar with lid.

Morning Wake-Up Body Cleanser

This refreshing and deodorizing blend will leave you clean and ready to start the day.

Blend:

8 ounces unscented liquid body soap.

12 drops peppermint

12 drops tangerine

6 drops coriander

Directions:

Pour oils into bottle containing liquid soap. Shake to mix.

Apply to loofah in shower.

Vanilla-Scented Body Moisturizer

This thick, creamy blend will leave your skin soft and smooth.

Blend:

20 drops vanilla

20 drops lavender or rose

2 ounces cocoa butter

2 ounces coconut oil

1 ounce avocado oil

Directions:

Cream together the cocoa butter with the coconut and avocado oils until well blended. Add in the essential oils and mix well.

Store mixture in glass jar with lid.

Dandruff Shampoo

This shampoo blend will help relieve dry scalp and flaking.

Blend:

4 ounces unscented shampoo

20 drops rose

15 drops carrot

10 drops rosemary

10 drops palmarosa

10 drops sandalwood

Directions:

Combine all ingredients together in bottle. Mix well.

Home and Yard

Essential oils can also be used around the home for a variety of purposes. Use as air freshener, insect repellant, and cleaners.

Air Freshening Room Spray

This blend has disinfecting properties as well as smelling terrific.

Blend:

4 ounces distilled water

20 drops lemon

15 drops bergamot

10 drops thyme

5 drops ylang ylang

Directions:

Combine ingredients in a clean spray bottle. Mist lightly in room.

To use as a vacuum refresher, place on cotton balls and leave in vacuum canister.

Bug Repellant

Follow this simple recipe to make an at home alternative to commercial bug repellants.

Blend:

4 ounces distilled water

15 drops citronella

10 drops geranium

10 drops eucalyptus

5 drops lemongrass

Directions:

Pour distilled water into a spray bottle. Add essential oils and shake well to mix.

Spritz onto skin and clothing.

Shake well between applications.

Multi-Purpose Cleaner

Use as a natural alternative to harsh chemical cleaners.

Blend:

8 ounces distilled water

1/2 teaspoon liquid castile soap

25 drops lemon

25 drops eucalyptus

Directions:

Pour distilled water into a spray bottle. Add essential oils and shake well to mix.

Pets

Pets can also benefit from essential oils! Like humans, dogs can also be sensitive to essential oils so always do a patch test and wait 24-48 hours to check for reaction.

Anti-Anxiety Blend for Pets

This will help to calm dogs suffering from separation anxiety.

Blend:

10 drops lavender

6 drops valerian

6 drops marjoram

4 drops clary sage

1 ounce carrier oil

Directions:

Rub 3-4 drops (more on larger size dogs or those with thick coats) of the blend into dogs fur concentrating on the ears, feet, chest, and inner legs.

Flea and Tick Repellant

Use this flea and tick repellant to deter pests and keep your pet smelling great.

Blend:

4 ounces distilled water

8 drops lemongrass

8 drops eucalyptus

8 drops lavender

Directions:

Combine ingredients in spray bottle. Shake well to mix.

Mist on pet's fur lightly. Repeat as needed.

Essential Oils for Beginners

Index of Symptoms

- **Abdominal cramps**: blue cypress; calendula; clove; peppermint; Roman chamomile
- **Acne**: benzoin; bergamot; cajeput; camphor; cedarwood; clove; galbanum; geranium; goldenrod; helichrysum; juniper; lemon; litsea cubeba; lovage leaf; mandarin; myrtle; palmarosa; petitgrain; Roman chamomile; tansy; tea tree
- **Addiction**: bergamot
- **Adrenal fatigue**: nutmeg
- **Allergies**: blue tansy; Roman chamomile
- **Amenorrhea**: bay laurel
- **Anemia**: carrot seed
- **Anger**: bergamot; davana; neroli; petitgrain; rose; vetiver
- **Anxiety**: allspice; angelica; balsam fir; bergamot; catnip; cedarwood; clary sage; coriander; frankincense; German chamomile; hinoki; ho wood; hops; hyssop; juniper; lavandin; lavender; lemon balm; neroli; patchouli; petitgrain; rose; sandalwood; spikenard; St. John's wort; valerian; vanilla; vetiver; ylang ylang
- **Aphrodisiacs**: amyris; clary sage; neroli; orange; patchouli; rosewood; vanilla
- **Appetite**: bitter orange; black pepper; ginger; mace

- **Arthritis:** allspice; bay laurel; benzoin; black spruce; camphor; cardamom; cedarwood; celery seed; cilantro; cistus; clove; ginger; Idaho blue spruce; mace; oregano; pine; St. John's wort; tumeric
- **Asthma:** balsam fir; bay laurel; benzoin; blue tansy; cajeput; celery seed; clove; frankincense; hinoki; Roman chamomile
- **Athlete's foot:** blue cypress; grapefruit; lemongrass; manuka; myrrh; tea tree
- **Bad breath:** cardamom; clove; mace
- **Bloating:** bay laurel; davana; juniper; ledum; litsea cubeba; rosemary
- **Blood sugar:** cinnamon; coriander; davana; dill
- **Boils:** bergamot; cistus; galbanum; German chamomile; myrrh; niaouli
- **Bronchitis:** allspice; anise seed; balsam fir; basil; bay laurel; benzoin; cajeput; camphor; clove; copaiba; fir needle; frankincense; hinoki; Idaho blue spruce; sandalwood; tagetes
- **Bruises:** helichrysum; lavender; Roman chamomile; tansy
- **Burns:** carrot seed; clove; fir needle; geranium; German chamomile; lavender; St. John's wort; tea tree
- **Calming:** allspice; clary sage; davana; lavender; petitgrain; vanilla
- **Candida.** *see* Yeast infections
- **Cardiovascular health:** celery seed; fennel; lavender; palmarosa; tansy; ylang ylang

- **Cellulite**: cypress; grapefruit; lemon; lime; rosemary
- **Chills**: black pepper; fir needle; ginger
- **Circulation**: Bay West Indies; benzoin; black pepper; cilantro; cinnamon; cistus; cypress; galbanum; grapefruit; mace; nutmeg; rose
- **Cold sores**: bergamot; blue cypress; geranium; manuka; myrrh
- **Colds**: anise seed; balsam fir; basil; bay laurel; Bay West Indies; benzoin; black pepper; cajeput; camphor; cilantro; cinnamon; cistus; dorado azil; frankincense; ginger; grapefruit; ledum; lemon; lemongrass; lime; litsea cubeba; tea tree
- **Colic**: cajeput; cardamom; carrot seed; cilantro; fennel; ginger; mountain savory; Roman chamomile
- **Colitis**: clove; geranium; neroli; peppermint
- **Concentration**: peppermint; rosemary; thyme
- **Congestion**: cedarwood; elemi; ginger; hinoki; ledum; marjoram; myrtle; tagetes
- **Constipation**: carrot seed; copaiba; dill; lemon; mace; orange; tangerine; yarrow
- **Coughs**: allspice; anise seed; balsam fir; basil; benzoin; camphor; cardamom; cinnamon; cistus; dorado azil; elemi; fir needle; frankincense; ginger; hinoki; jasmine; ledum; lemongrass; myrtle; sandalwood; tagetes
- **Cramps**: catnip; coriander; galbanum; ginger; hops; mountain savory; Roman chamomile; tumeric; yarrow

- **Cuts and scrapes:** galbanum; Idaho blue spruce; St. John's wort; yarrow
- **Cystitis:** cedarwood; celery seed; clove; niaouli
- **Dandruff:** basil; Bay West Indies; cedarwood; juniper; manuka; rosemary; sage
- **Dark spots:** mandarin
- **Decongestant:** amyris; hyssop; Idaho blue spruce; patchouli
- **Dental infections:** Bay West Indies
- **Depression:** allspice; basil; benzoin; bergamot; birch; camphor; clary sage; davana; frankincense; grapefruit; ho wood; jasmine; lavandin; lavender; lemon balm; Melissa; neroli; orange; patchouli; peppermint; petitgrain; rose; rosewood; sandalwood; thyme; valerian; vanilla; ylang ylang
- **Dermatitis:** carrot seed; cistus; German chamomile; lovage leaf; palmarosa; Roman chamomile; tansy
- **Detoxification:** catnip; cilantro; coriander; juniper
- **Diabetes:** cinnamon; davana
- **Diarrhea:** Bay West Indies; black pepper; carrot seed; cilantro; copaiba; ginger; mountain savory; neroli; tangerine
- **Digestive complaints:** allspice; bay laurel; black pepper; cajeput; celery seed; cilantro; cinnamon; davana; dill; fennel; ginger; juniper; mountain savory; neroli; spearmint; tangerine; tarragon; tumeric
- **Dry skin:** blue cypress; carrot seed; German chamomile; myrrh; oak moss; patchouli; Roman cham-

omile
- **Eczema**: benzoin; bergamot; blue cypress; carrot seed; cedarwood; cistus; geranium; German chamomile; juniper; lemon balm; lovage leaf; Roman chamomile; sandalwood
- **Edema**: bay laurel; carrot seed; cypress; lovage leaf
- **Endometriosis**: eucalyptus
- **Fatigue**: angelica; basil; cilantro; lemongrass; peppermint; pine; thyme
- **Fear**: bergamot; rose; sandalwood; ylang ylang
- **Fever**: basil; black pepper; cajeput; eucalyptus; fir needle; ginger; ledum; lime; niaouli
- **Fibroids**: cistus
- **Flatulence**: anise seed; basil; cardamom; cilantro; cornmint; fennel; myrrh
- **Flu**: anise seed; balsam fir; bay laurel; Bay West Indies; black pepper; camphor; cilantro; cinnamon; cistus; eucalyptus; ginger; ledum; lime; tea tree
- **Fungal infections**: black pepper; geranium; mandarin; manuka; myrrh; patchouli; tea tree
- **Gallbladder**: carrot seed
- **Gas**: bay laurel; davana; dill; fennel
- **Gastric pain**: Roman chamomile
- **Gingivitis**: myrrh; rose
- **Gout**: angelica; basil; cajeput; carrot seed; celery seed; juniper; nutmeg; tansy
- **Hair growth**: Bay West Indies; grapefruit; rosemary; ylang ylang
- **Hair loss**: cedarwood
- **Halitosis**: cardamom; clove; mace

- **Headache:** basil; cajeput; cardamom; eucalyptus; lavandin; lemongrass; oregano; peppermint; rosemary; St. John's wort
- **Heart palpitations:** clary sage; neroli
- **Heartburn:** black pepper; cardamom
- **Hemorrhoids:** cistus; copaiba; cypress; fir needle; geranium; myrrh; St. John's wort; yarrow
- **Herpes blisters:** geranium; lemon
- **Hiccups:** dill; fennel; tarragon
- **Hoarseness:** jasmine
- **Hormone balance:** clary sage; davana; fennel; geranium; myrtle; rose; sage
- **Hot flashes:** clary sage
- **Hypertension:** celery seed; clove; lemon balm; rose; tansy; ylang ylang
- **Immune system:** cistus; eucalyptus; lemon; lime; orange; ravensara; tansy
- **Impotence:** goldenrod; jasmine; nutmeg; rose
- **Indigestion:** allspice; cardamom; cornmint; ginger; hops; hyssop; mountain savory
- **Infection:** balsam fir; bay laurel; bergamot; blue cypress; camphor; cilantro; hyssop; Idaho blue spruce; lemon; lemon myrtle; lime; ravensara; tea tree
- **Infertility:** sage
- **Inflammation:** bergamot; blue tansy; camphor; cinnamon; clary sage; galbanum; hyssop; lavandin; lavender; lemongrass; nutmeg; tumeric
- **Insect bites and stings:** basil; bergamot; cajeput; copaiba; lavender; niaouli; patchouli; sage
- **Insect repellant:** basil; blue cypress; camphor; cat-

nip; citronella; lemon balm; litsea cubeba; palo santo; tagetes; tansy
- **Insomnia:** basil; catnip; clary sage; German chamomile; hops; lavender; lemon balm; mandarin; neroli; petitgrain; sandalwood; spikenard; valerian; vanilla; vetiver
- **Itching:** cedarwood; lavender; manuka; patchouli; Roman chamomile; sandalwood
- **Kidney problems:** celery seed; ledum; spruce; tansy
- **Laryngitis:** cajeput; jasmine; ledum; niaouli
- **Lice:** geranium
- **Liver tonic:** bay laurel; blue tansy; carrot seed; geranium; German chamomile; goldenrod; grapefruit; helichrysum; ledum
- **Lymphatic system:** blue tansy; cypress; grapefruit; lemon; sandalwood
- **Menopause:** clary sage; galbanum; geranium; German chamomile; sage
- **Menstrual problems:** cistus; clary sage; cypress; geranium; German chamomile; juniper; lovage leaf; marjoram; myrrh; nutmeg; parsley seed; rose; sage; tarragon; yarrow
- **Mental fatigue:** basil; cardamom; coriander; hyssop; jasmine; pine; rosemary; spearmint
- **Migraine:** basil; cilantro; German chamomile; lemon balm; rosemary; spikenard
- **Molluscum contagiosum:** lemon myrtle; tea tree
- **Morning sickness:** ginger
- **Motion sickness:** ginger
- **Mouth ulcers:** benzoin; clove; cornmint

- **Muscle aches and pains:** allspice; anise seed; balsam fir; basil; Bay West Indies; benzoin; black pepper; black spruce; blue cypress; blue tansy; camphor; cilantro; cinnamon; galbanum; ginger; grapefruit; jasmine; mace; nutmeg; oregano; pine; St. John's wort; tumeric; vetiver
- **Muscle relaxant:** amyris; angelica; catnip
- **Muscle spasms:** petitgrain
- **Nausea:** allspice; black pepper; cajeput; cardamom; cilantro; cornmint; fennel; ginger; mountain savory; peppermint; tumeric
- **Nervous tension:** allspice; catnip; cedarwood; cistus; German chamomile; goldenrod; hinoki; ho wood; hops; jasmine; juniper; lavandin; lavender; marjoram; neroli; petitgrain; rose; sandalwood; spikenard; St. John's wort; valerian; vanilla; vetiver; ylang ylang
- **Neuralgia:** allspice; Bay West Indies
- **Night sweats:** clary sage
- **Nosebleeds:** cypress
- **Oily skin:** Bay West Indies; carrot seed; cedarwood; fennel; juniper; lemon; litsea cubeba; mandarin; myrtle; petitgrain
- **Pain relief:** balsam fir; black pepper; blue tansy; cajeput; clove; hops; oregano
- **Panic attacks:** petitgrain; valerian; ylang ylang
- **Parasites:** clove; davana; fir needle; hyssop; mountain savory; niaouli; oregano; tarragon
- **Premature ejaculation:** jasmine
- **Premenstrual syndrome (PMS):** clary sage; galba-

num; geranium; lavender; Roman chamomile; tarragon
- **Prostate**: myrrh; myrtle
- **Psoriasis**: angelica; benzoin; bergamot; cajeput; carrot seed; German chamomile; juniper
- **Rashes**: benzoin; blue cypress; cajeput; carrot seed; German chamomile; palmarosa; Roman chamomile; spikenard
- **Relaxation**: anise seed; catnip; frankincense; German chamomile; petitgrain
- **Respiratory infections**: anise seed; dorado azil; Douglas fir; elemi; eucalyptus; hyssop; sandalwood; spruce
- **Rheumatism**: allspice; balsam fir; basil; bay laurel; Bay West Indies; benzoin; black pepper; black spruce; cajeput; camphor; carrot seed; cedarwood; celery seed; cilantro; cinnamon; frankincense; Idaho blue spruce; oregano; pine; tumeric
- **Ringworm**: blue cypress; geranium; manuka; myrrh
- **Scalp conditions**: Bay West Indies; manuka; rosemary; ylang ylang
- **Scars**: benzoin; carrot seed; cistus; frankincense; helichrysum; lavender; mandarin; palmarosa; patchouli; sandalwood
- **Sciatica**: balsam fir; blue tansy; cardamom; sandalwood; St. John's wort; tansy; tarragon
- **Sexual dysfunction**: jasmine; nutmeg
- **Shingles**: geranium; mountain savory; ravensara
- **Sinusitis**: balsam fir; basil; cajeput; cardamom;

cedarwood; clove; eucalyptus; niaouli; ravensara
- **Skin conditions:** Bay West Indies; benzoin; bergamot; blue cypress; blue tansy; cajeput; carrot seed; cedarwood; galbanum; geranium; German chamomile; juniper; lavender; lovage leaf; mandarin; manuka; myrtle; patchouli; Roman chamomile; tansy
- **Sore throat:** benzoin; cajeput; copaiba; fir needle; ginger; myrrh; myrtle; oregano; Roman chamomile
- **Spasms:** catnip; valerian
- **Sprains:** blue tansy; ginger; jasmine
- **Stress:** angelica; anise seed; balsam fir; benzoin; bergamot; blue tansy; coriander; cypress; davana; grapefruit; ho wood; hops; juniper; lavender; lemongrass; mandarin; patchouli; peppermint; petitgrain; rose; sandalwood; spikenard; St. John's wort; valerian; vetiver; ylang ylang
- **Stretch marks:** galbanum; helichrysum; lavandin; neroli
- **Sunburn:** blue tansy; carrot seed; lavender; St. John's wort
- **Teething pain:** German chamomile; Roman chamomile
- **Tension:** balsam fir; benzoin; clary sage; coriander; frankincense; grapefruit; jasmine; marjoram
- **Tonsillitis:** oregano
- **Tooth ache:** cajeput; clove; German chamomile; lavandin; tansy
- **Ulcer:** bergamot; cinnamon; rose; sage
- **Urinary tract infection:** balsam fir; bergamot; cedarwood; celery seed; copaiba; mountain savory;

tarragon
- **Vaginal infections:** eucalyptus; mountain savory
- **Varicose veins:** bergamot; cypress; St. John's wort; vanilla; yarrow
- **Viral infections:** bay laurel; black spruce; blue cypress; cinnamon; hyssop; Idaho blue spruce
- **Vomiting:** cajeput; cardamom; fennel
- **Warts:** cinnamon; helichrysum
- **Water retention:** angelica; carrot seed; cypress; grapefruit; hyssop; juniper; tangerine
- **Weight loss:** bitter orange; grapefruit; ledum; orange
- **Wounds:** balsam fir; benzoin; bergamot; black spruce; carrot seed; cistus; dill; fir needle; geranium; helichrysum; myrrh; niaouli; oak moss; patchouli; rose; tagetes; tea tree; yarrow
- **Wrinkles:** carrot seed; cistus; fennel; galbanum; helichrysum; mandarin; myrrh; neroli; palmarosa; patchouli; rose
- **Yeast infections:** blue cypress; palmarosa; peppermint; rosemary

Essential Oils for Beginners

Conclusion

Over the centuries, essential oils have been used in many different ways. Some have become popular as cures to common ailments, and others are loved simply for their smell and stress relieving properties. One common thread remains, however, we will continue to discover new uses for these amazing oils.

You now have enough information to start experimenting with how essential oils can benefit you and your family. I have no doubt that you will find them beneficial in a multitude of ways.

It's okay to start slowly, using just one or two essential oils at a time. As your experience grows, so will your repertoire.

Have fun and be healthy!

Essential Oils for Beginners

Resources and References

Books on Essential Oils and Aromatherapy

For more information on aromatherapy and essential oils check out these sources of information.

- *375 Essential Oils and Hydrosols* by Jeanne Rose
- *Advanced Aromatherapy* by Kurt Schnaubelt
- *Aromatherapy for the Healthy Child* by Valerie Ann Wormwood
- *The Art of Aromatherapy* by Robert Tisserand
- *The Complete Book Essential Oils & Aromatherapy* by Valerie Ann Worwood
- *Essential Oil Safety: A Guide for Health Care Practitioners* by Robert Tisserand and Tony Balacs
- *The Essential Oils Book* by Colleen K. Dodt

- *Holistic Aromatherapy for Animals* by Kristen Leigh Bell
- *Hydrosols: The Next Aromatherapy* by Suzanne Catty
- *The Illustrated Encyclopedia of Essential Oils* by Julia Lawless
- *Practical Aromatherapy: How to Use Essential Oils to Restore Vitality* by Shirley Price

Sources of Essential Oils

Here are a list of recommended sources for purchasing essential oils and other supplies.

Arlys Naturals

All natural essential oils and skin care products.

www.arlysnaturals.com

1-877-502-7597

Artisan Aromatics

Tests each essential oil for quality assurance.

http://ArtisanEssentialOils.com

1-828-835-2231

Liberty Natural Products

Grower, importer, and wholesaler.

www.libertynatural.com

1-800-289-8427

Mountain Rose Herbs

Established in 1987.

www.mountainroseherbs.com

1-800-879-3337

Essential Oils for Beginners

From the Author

Thank you for reading *Essential Oils for Beginners*. I sincerely hope that you found this book informative and helpful.

It would be greatly appreciated if you could take a few moments to share your opinion and post a review for this book. Your positive review helps us to reach other readers and provides valuable feedback with which we can improve future books.

Thank you!

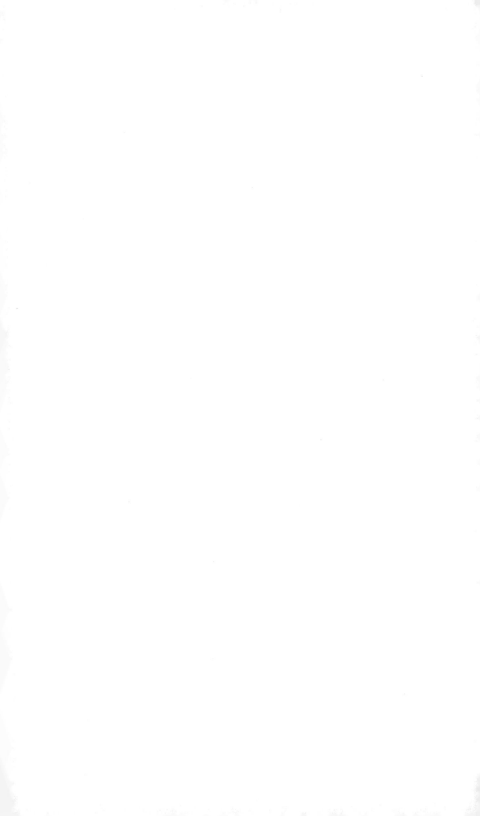

Made in the USA
Middletown, DE
10 March 2015